Economic & Social Affairs

World Fertility Report 2013: Fertility at the Extremes

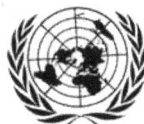

United Nations

This page is intentionally left blank

ST/ESA/SER.A/331

Department of Economic and Social Affairs
Population Division

World Fertility Report 2013: Fertility at the Extremes

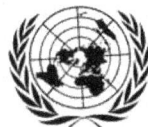

United Nations
New York, 2014

DESA

The Department of Economic and Social Affairs of the United Nations Secretariat is a vital interface between global policies in the economic, social and environmental spheres and national action. The Department works in three main interlinked areas: (i) it compiles, generates and analyses a wide range of economic, social and environmental data and information on which States Members of the United Nations draw to review common problems and take stock of policy options; (ii) it facilitates the negotiations of Member States in many intergovernmental bodies on joint courses of action to address ongoing or emerging global challenges; and (iii) it advises interested Governments on the ways and means of translating policy frameworks developed in United Nations conferences and summits into programmes at the country level and, through technical assistance, helps build national capacities.

Note

The designations employed in this report and the material presented in it do not imply the expression of any opinion whatsoever on the part of the Secretariat of the United Nations concerning the legal status of any country, territory, city or area or of its authorities, or concerning the delimitation of its frontiers or boundaries.

This publication has been issued without formal editing.

Suggested citation:
United Nations, Department of Economic and Social Affairs, Population Division (2014). *World Fertility Report 2013: Fertility at the Extremes* (United Nations publication).

ST/ESA/SER.A/331

UNITED NATIONS PUBLICATION

PREFACE

The Population Division of the Department of Economic and Social Affairs of the United Nations Secretariat is responsible for providing the international community with up-to-date and impartial information on population and development. The Population Division provides guidance on population and development issues to the United Nations General Assembly, the Economic and Social Council and the Commission on Population and Development, and undertakes regular studies on population estimates and projections, fertility, mortality, migration, reproductive health, population policies and population and development interrelationships.

As part of its work on fertility, the Population Division monitors levels and trends in age and parity patterns of fertility and its proximate determinants, such as marriage and contraceptive use, collects and analyses information on the relationship between fertility and development, and provides substantive support to intergovernmental discussions at the United Nations on the topics of fertility, family planning and development.

World Fertility Report 2013: Fertility at the Extremes is the fifth in a series and focuses on trends in fertility over the past 20 years and key factors underlying these trends for countries at the extremes of fertility: 66 countries with more than 3.2 children per woman in 2005-2010 and 70 countries with 2.0 children per woman or less in 2005-2010. The data presented are from *World Population Prospects: The 2012 Revision*, the official United Nations publication of population estimates and projections. Country data are taken from the same report, other United Nations sources or national sources, as appropriate.

This report was prepared by Ms. Petra Nahmias with substantive inputs from Mr. Stephen Kisambira and Ms. Ann Biddlecom. Ms. Donna Culpepper and Ms. Natalia Devyatkin provided editorial support. Ms. Francesca Perucci reviewed and provided helpful comments on the draft report.

The *World Fertility Report* series as well as other population information may be accessed on the Population Division's website at www.unpopulation.org. For further information concerning this publication, please contact the office of the Director, Population Division, Department of Economic and Social Affairs, United Nations, New York, 10017, USA, telephone (212) 963-3209, fax (212) 963-2147, email: population@un.org

CONTENTS

PREFACE iii
EXPLANATORY NOTES vii
KEY FINDINGS viii

INTRODUCTION 1

Chapter
    I.   LOW FERTILITY 3
          A. The transition to below-replacement fertility 5
          B. Fertility decline at young and old ages 7
          C. Completed fertility and childlessness 13
          D. Childbearing and marriage 15
          E. Fertility projections 20
          F. Consequences of low fertility 21
          G. Policy approaches to low fertility 22

    II.   HIGH FERTILITY 27
          A. Changes in total fertility and age-specific fertility rates 27
          B. Fertility projections 36
          C. Changes in fertility timing, marriage and contraceptive use 37
          D. Fertility decline and socio-economic development 43
          E. Consequences of high fertility 47
          F. Policy approaches to high fertility 48

CONCLUSION 52

REFERENCES 53

ANNEXES 61

FIGURES

I.1.   Levels of total fertility in low-fertility countries, 2005-2010 4
I.2.   Trends in total fertility among current low-fertility countries, 1950-2010 6
I.3.   Adolescent birth rate in 1990-1995 and 2005-2010 and adolescent birth rate
        as a percentage of total fertility in 2005-2010, low-fertility countries 8
I.4.   Mean age at first birth, around 1994 and latest point available, low-fertility countries 9
I.5.   Number of births per 1,000 women aged 40-44, 1990-1995 and 2005-2010, low-fertility countries 10
I.6.   Proportion of total fertility attributable to births to women aged 40-44, 1990-1995 and
        2005-2010, low-fertility countries 11
I.7.   Age-specific fertility rates among low-fertility countries by region, 2005-2010 12
I.8.   Percentage of women aged 40-44 who are childless, around 1994 and latest point available,
        low-fertility countries 14
I.9.   Percentage of women aged 40-44 who are childless or with three or more children, latest
        point available, low-fertility countries 15
I.10.   Percentage of births outside of marriage, around 1994 and latest point available, low-fertility
        countries 16
I.11.   Female mean age at first marriage, around 1994 and latest point available, low-fertility countries 18
I.12.   Percentage of women aged 40-44 who never married, around 1994 and latest point available,
        low-fertility countries 19

I.13. Total fertility for countries by major area, estimates for 2005-2010 and projections for 2030-2035, low-fertility countries 20

I.14. Old-age dependency ratio, 1995 to 2035, low-fertility countries 22

I.15. Percentage of low-fertility countries with government policies on fertility levels by type of policy, 1996 and 2013 23

II.1. Levels of total fertility in high-fertility countries, 2005-2010 28

II.2. Maximum fertility and onset of fertility decline among high-fertility countries 29

II.3. Fertility decline in high-fertility countries from 1994 to 2010 31

II.4. Adolescent birth rates in 1990-1995 and 2005-2010, high-fertility countries 32

II.5. Birth rate of women aged 40-44 in 1990-1995 and 2005-2010, high-fertility countries 33

II.6. Percentage change in the birth rates of adolescents and women aged 40-44 between 1990-1995 and 2005-2010, high-fertility countries 34

II.7. Percentage decline in total fertility attributed to change in birth rates among women aged 15-19 and 40-44, 1990-1995 to 2005-2010, high-fertility countries 36

II.8. Total fertility for countries, 2005-2010 and projections for 2030-2035, high-fertility countries 37

II.9. Adolescent birth rate and mean age at first marriage and first birth, selected high-fertility countries, 1990s to latest data available.. 39

II.10. Contraceptive prevalence rate in 1994 and 2014, high-fertility countries 40

II.11. Change in total fertility between 1990-1995 and 2005-2010 and change in contraceptive prevalence rate between 1994 and 2010, high-fertility countries 41

II.12. Unmet need for limiting and for spacing, latest data available, high-fertility countries 43

II.13. Proportion of urban population and years of school life expectancy for females among high-fertility countries in the quartiles with longest and shortest durations between the timing of peak fertility and the onset of fertility transition, high-fertility countries 45

II.14. Infant mortality and contraceptive prevalence among high-fertility countries in the quartiles with longest and shortest durations between the timing of peak fertility and onset of the fertility transition, high-fertility countries 46

II.15. Percentage of high-fertility countries with government policies on fertility levels by type of policy, 1996 and 2013 49

ANNEX TABLES

1. Indicators and data sources 61

2. Female mean age at first birth around 1994 and the most recent year, low-fertility countries with data for both periods... 62

3. Completed fertility: Women aged 40-44 childless and with three or more children, low-fertility countries with data for both periods 63

4. Percentage of births outside marriage, around 1994 and the most recent year, low-fertility countries with data for both periods 65

5. Maximum fertility between 1950 and 2010 and onset of fertility transition in high-fertility countries 66

6. Decline in total fertility in high-fertility countries between 1994 and 2010 67

7. Female mean age at first marriage and age at first birth around 1994 and the most recent year, high-fertility countries with data for both periods 68

EXPLANATORY NOTES

The following symbols have been used in the tables throughout this report:

Two dots (..) indicate that data are not available or are not reported separately.
A hyphen (-) indicates that the item is not applicable.
A minus sign (-) before a figure indicates a decrease.
A full stop (.) is used to indicate decimals.
Use of a hyphen (-) between years, for example, 1995-2000, signifies the full period involved.

Numbers and percentages in tables do not necessarily add to totals because of rounding.

References to countries, territories and areas:

The designations employed and the material in this publication do not imply the expression of any opinion whatsoever on the part of the Secretariat of the United Nations concerning the legal status of any country, territory or area or its authorities, or concerning the delimitation of its frontiers or boundaries.

The term "country" as used in this publication also refers, as appropriate, to territories or areas.

Names and compositions of geographical areas follow those of "Standard country or area codes for statistical use" (ST/ESA/STAT/SER.M/49/Rev.3), available at http://unstats.un.org/unsd/methods/m49/m49.htm.

KEY FINDINGS

- Fertility has declined significantly since the 1994 International Conference on Population and Development, yet 66 countries remain with high fertility levels (more than 3.2 children per woman). The number of low-fertility countries (with 2.0 children per woman or less) has increased from 51 countries at the time of the 1994 ICPD to 70 countries today.

- High-fertility countries are increasingly concentrated in sub-Saharan Africa (45 out of 66 high-fertility countries) while low-fertility countries are becoming more diverse geographically, including many more countries in Asia and Latin America and the Caribbean (31 out of the 70 low-fertility countries are from regions outside of Europe).

- There have been substantial declines in adolescent fertility in many high-fertility countries, but adolescent fertility remains very high in Middle Africa and Western Africa. Angola, Chad, Mali and Niger stand out with adolescent birth rates of above 180 births per 1,000 women aged 15-19 years in 2005-2010. Adolescent fertility also continues to account for a high proportion of births in many low-fertility countries in Latin America and the Caribbean; in five low-fertility countries, all in Latin America and the Caribbean, 15 per cent or more of all births were to adolescent mothers.

- Fertility is projected to decrease in high-fertility countries. Some of these countries, especially in Asia, are projected to experience a sharp decline. The fertility decline in other countries is projected to be more gradual with Mali and Niger standing out as remaining with particularly high fertility. Among high-fertility countries, 16 are projected to reach total fertility of 2.6 or below by 2030-2035. All 17 countries with projected fertility of 3.8 or more are in Eastern, Middle and Western Africa.

- Most low-fertility countries are projected to increase their fertility or for it to remain relatively stable to 2030-2035 (52 out of 70 countries). The greatest increase is projected to be in the lowest fertility countries: 18 countries, all with a total fertility of less than 1.5 in 2005-2010, are projected to increase total fertility by 0.3 children per woman or more by 2030-2035.

- The female mean age at first birth has increased in both low-fertility and high-fertility countries. However, the age at first birth remains young in many high-fertility countries, especially in sub-Saharan Africa where nine of the countries with available data report a mean age at first birth of below 19 years. In many low-fertility countries, the postponement of first birth to older ages is becoming more common, with four countries (Greece, Italy, Luxembourg and Switzerland) reporting a mean age at first birth of 30 years or older whereas no countries had reached this level around 1994.

- In low-fertility countries, there has been an increase in childlessness among women aged 40-44 years, especially in Eastern Asia and Europe, with five countries reaching a level of childlessness where more than one woman in five has no children by the age of 40-44 years, a level not seen in any country around 1994. There has also been an increase in childbearing outside of marriage in low-fertility countries and areas with more than half of children currently born outside of marriage in Martinique, Norway, Puerto Rico and Sweden.

- In high-fertility countries, there has been a dramatic increase in the contraceptive prevalence rate, especially in Eastern Africa where it more than doubled in 13 out of 16 high-fertility countries, in some cases increasing more than tenfold. Despite this increase, high levels of unmet need for family planning remain, with more than one married woman in four having an unmet need in half of the high-fertility countries. Most unmet need for family planning in the high-fertility countries of Africa is for delaying or spacing births whereas in the high-fertility countries of Asia and Latin America and the Caribbean most unmet need for family planning is for stopping childbearing (i.e., women wish to have no more children).

- High-fertility countries will be faced with a growing and youthful population, even with further fertility declines in the future. There are opportunities to benefit from changes in the age structure brought about by continued declines in fertility if increased investments in human capital, job growth and other supportive policies are put in place.

- Most low-fertility countries will experience population ageing although the extent will depend on how long a country has experienced low fertility and how low fertility has declined. The changing age structure will present a challenge especially for the increasing number of low-fertility middle-income countries.

INTRODUCTION

Fertility patterns in the world have changed dramatically over the last two decades since the International Conference on Population and Development (ICPD) in 1994, producing a world with very diverse childbearing patterns. Further complicating this picture are questions regarding the future path that fertility change will take in countries experiencing high levels or low levels of childbearing and the effective policy approaches to address population and development implications of these diverse childbearing patterns.

The *World Fertility Report 2013: Fertility at the Extremes*, the fifth in a series, adopts a particular focus on countries where fertility levels are high (more than 3.2 children per woman) and countries where fertility levels are low (2.0 children per woman or less). In 1990-1995, around the time of the ICPD, 105 countries had high fertility as opposed to just 66 countries in 2005-2010 (the period of the most recent fertility estimates). Several countries, such as Iran, the United Arab Emirates and Viet Nam, experienced rapid fertility declines over this time period, moving from high fertility to low fertility over the span of a single generation. High-fertility countries are increasingly concentrated in sub-Saharan Africa while low-fertility countries have moved from being predominantly European to include countries from Asia and Latin America and the Caribbean.

What have been the pathways countries have taken that resulted in levels of fertility at the extremes of today? How have key correlates of fertility changed over time and how similar are the patterns in these correlates for countries at high or low fertility levels? What are the social and economic consequences and policy approaches for countries with fertility at the extremes? This report addresses these questions drawing on a long time series of fertility estimates and updated data from countries on selected correlates of fertility change. Available policy options are also discussed.

For the purposes of this report, 66 countries are categorized as high fertility (i.e., countries or areas with total fertility of more than 3.2 children per woman in 2005-2010) and 70 countries are categorized as low fertility (i.e., countries or areas with total fertility of 2.0 children per woman or less in 2005-2010).[1] Estimates and projections of total fertility and age-specific fertility rates were taken from the 2012 Revision of *World Population Prospects* (United Nations, 2013a) to enable comparability over time and to include the maximum number of countries or areas in the analyses. Countries or areas[2] with at least 90,000 inhabitants in 2012 were included and are grouped geographically into six major areas (Africa, Asia, Europe, Latin America and the Caribbean, Northern America and Oceania) and 21 regions.

Data on other indicators of fertility and correlates of fertility change were taken from varied sources (see annex table 1). Model-based estimates of family planning indicators were drawn from a recent United Nations publication (United Nations, 2014a). Modelled data were not available for all indicators and thus estimates were drawn from a range of data sources, such as national censuses, national household surveys and vital registration. In these cases, the reference year is not the same but a short range of years was used for estimates around 1994 and for the latest point available. Information on national policies was obtained from the latest global assessment of population policies, based in part on official Government responses to the United Nations Inquiry among Governments on Population and Development.

---

[1] In previous editions of the *World Fertility Report*, analysis was also conducted by development group where countries were categorized as part of developed regions or developing regions. These development group categories were based on the fertility levels of countries around the 1960s (United Nations, 1966) and were not used in the present report because their meaning is increasingly ambiguous. Many countries classified as part of developing regions now have very low fertility (e.g., China) as well as high per capita income (e.g., the Republic of Korea and Singapore).
[2] The term "country" as used in this publication refers, as appropriate, to countries, territories or areas.

I. LOW FERTILITY

Low fertility (defined in this report as total fertility of 2.0 children per woman or less) is fast becoming the norm for many countries in the world and is no longer a predominantly European phenomenon. Countries in parts of Asia and Latin America and the Caribbean are experiencing fertility levels that are below the replacement level of 2.1 children per woman. Eastern Asia has become a region of especially low fertility, with total fertility of 1.4 children per woman or less in Hong Kong Special Administrative Region (SAR) of China, Japan, Macao SAR of China, and the Republic of Korea. While 39 of the 70 low-fertility countries in 2005-2010 are in Europe, 16 are in Asia and 12 are in Latin America and the Caribbean (figure I.1). Australia, Canada and Mauritius are the only low-fertility countries in Oceania, Northern America and Africa, respectively.

The transition to low fertility is occurring at faster rates and at lower levels of development than was traditionally seen in Europe and North America during their fertility transitions, meaning that fertility rates are converging at a faster pace than the convergence of many other socio-economic characteristics (Kohler and others, 2002). There is concern in many countries that, without migration, a rapid fertility transition poses serious challenges, including an expanding older population and a shrinking workforce to pay for social services and pensions and to drive economic growth. As more countries experience sustained low fertility, it is important to understand how countries differ in their trajectories toward low fertility and correlates of fertility change in order to inform effective policies that address the consequences of below-replacement fertility.

At the time of the 1994 ICPD, 51 of today's 70 low-fertility countries had fertility levels at 2.0 children per woman or less. This figure includes most low-fertility countries in Europe (figure I.2), which had already reached replacement-level fertility prior to the 1990s (Albania and the former Yugoslav Republic (TFYR) of Macedonia are exceptions to this pattern). In Eastern Asia, most low-fertility countries also reached below-replacement fertility before 1994, except in the Democratic People's Republic of Korea. Persistently low levels of fertility increasingly characterize countries in Eastern Asia, and the region has replaced Europe as the "global hotspot" of low fertility (Sobotka, 2013). Central Asia, Western Asia and Latin America and the Caribbean are emerging as new areas of low fertility. The majority of low-fertility countries in these regions did not have below-replacement fertility at the time of the 1994 ICPD.

Figure I.1. Levels of total fertility in low-fertility countries, 2005-2010

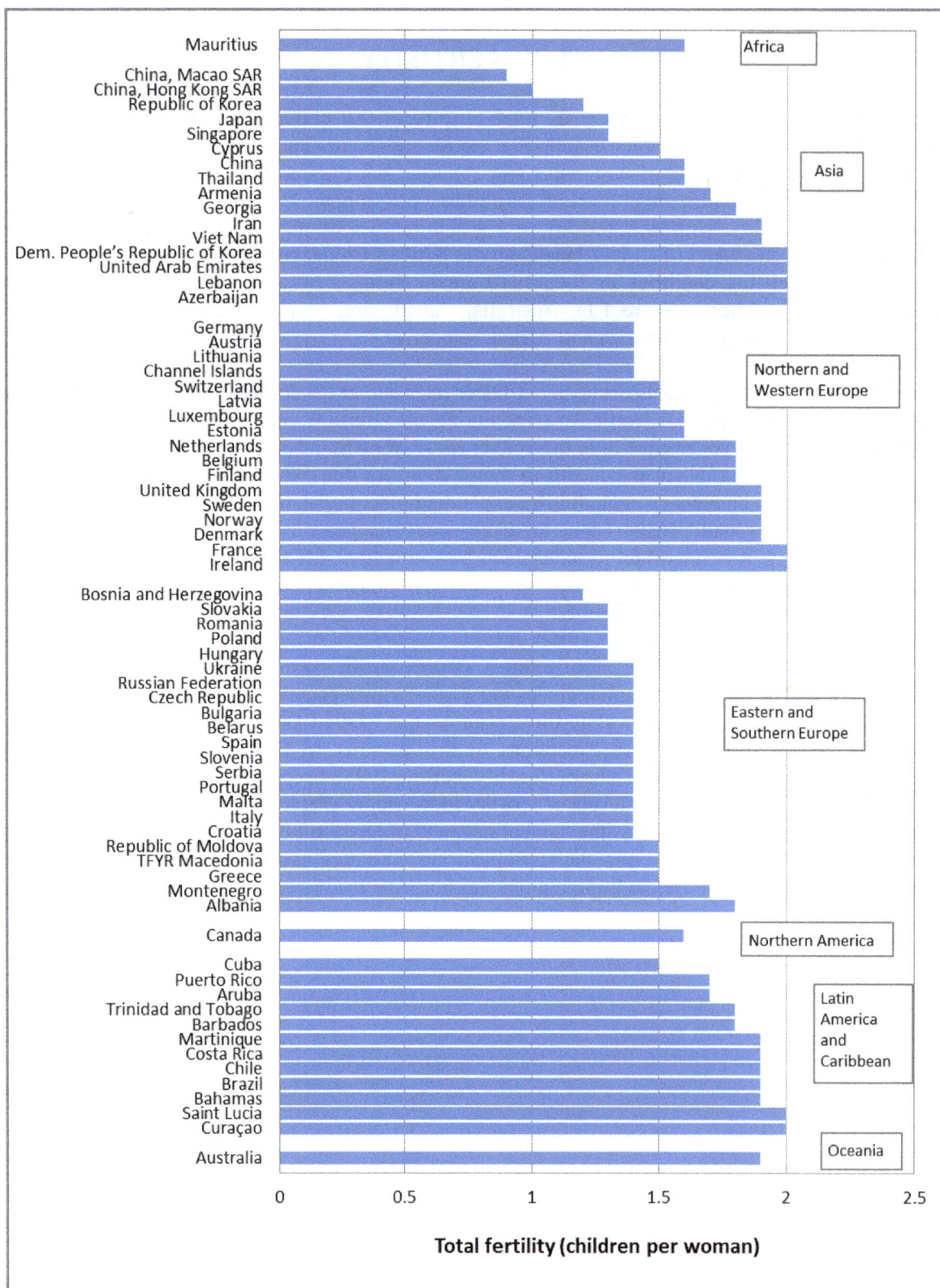

Total fertility (children per woman)

Source: United Nations (2013a).

A. THE TRANSITION TO BELOW-REPLACEMENT FERTILITY

Countries varied in the timing and speed of the transition to low fertility. The transition from the highest fertility level since 1950 to the lowest fertility level (figure I.2) was very steep in many countries, with the steepest transitions predominantly in regions outside of Europe. The maximum fertility reached since 1950 was much higher in the low-fertility countries of Asia and Latin America and the Caribbean than it was in Europe. Moreover, maximum fertility occurred much later in countries of Central Asia, Western Asia, and Latin America and the Caribbean compared to countries in other regions, followed by precipitous fertility declines within a short period. However, the most recent lowest fertility level reached in many countries in Central Asia, Western Asia, and Latin America and the Caribbean is still higher than that seen in other regions, suggesting that further decline in period total fertility is likely if current patterns continue. Costa Rica, Iran, Mauritius, Republic of Korea, Saint Lucia, Singapore, Thailand, Viet Nam and the United Arab Emirates stand out as having the most rapid rates of fertility decline per year (9 per cent to 11 per cent) since reaching maximum fertility. In Iran, for instance, total fertility declined from a maximum of 6.9 children per woman in 1960 to 1.9 children per woman in 2005; that is, a decline in total fertility of more than 1.1 children per woman per decade.

Total fertility was already below three children per woman in 1950 in the majority of European countries, and most reached maximum fertility (since 1950) below three children per woman between 1960 and 1970. Among countries that had a maximum total fertility of less than three children per woman in the 1960s or later, there is wide variation in the fertility trends though most reflect the "bump" of the baby boom period. Austria, Romania and Spain are among the five countries with both the highest and lowest period total fertility between 1960 and 2010, indicating that period total fertility declined rapidly in these countries at rates between 3 and 4 per cent per year. In Romania, in particular, the abolition of liberal abortion laws in 1966 led to a near doubling of fertility rates the following year (Berent, 1970).

Most countries that had a maximum total fertility of below three children per woman experienced the lowest dip in fertility around 2000, followed by an increase in fertility levels. By 2010, period total fertility was below 1.5 children per woman in all countries that experienced a maximum fertility level of less than 3.0 children per woman before 1960, except in France. Total fertility remained between 1.5 and 1.9 in most of the countries that had reached maximum fertility after 1960.

Half of the 22 countries or areas that had a maximum total fertility of three to five children per woman since 1950 were in Europe, five in Eastern Asia and Western Asia (Armenia, Cyprus, Democratic People's Republic of Korea, Georgia and Japan) and four in the Caribbean (Bahamas, Barbados, Cuba and Puerto Rico). The pattern of fertility trends in countries that reached maximum total fertility between three and five children per woman before 1960 shows rapid declines to around 1975, followed by stable trends from around 2000 to 2010.

In countries where maximum fertility occurred after 1960, there is a sharp decline between the maximum-fertility year and the onset of a stable total fertility level, beginning in 2002 in the Bahamas, 1991 in Ireland, 1980 in the Netherlands and 1990 in Portugal. Among these countries, the transition to relatively stable and low total fertility levels occurred earlier where maximum fertility was lower (Netherlands and Portugal) and later where maximum fertility was higher (Bahamas and Ireland).

Among the 22 countries that reached maximum period total fertility of above five children per woman since 1950, half were in Asia, eight in Latin America and the Caribbean, two in Europe and only one, Mauritius, in Africa. The majority of these countries reached maximum fertility in the 1950s.

Figure I.2. Trends in total fertility among current low-fertility countries, 1950-2010

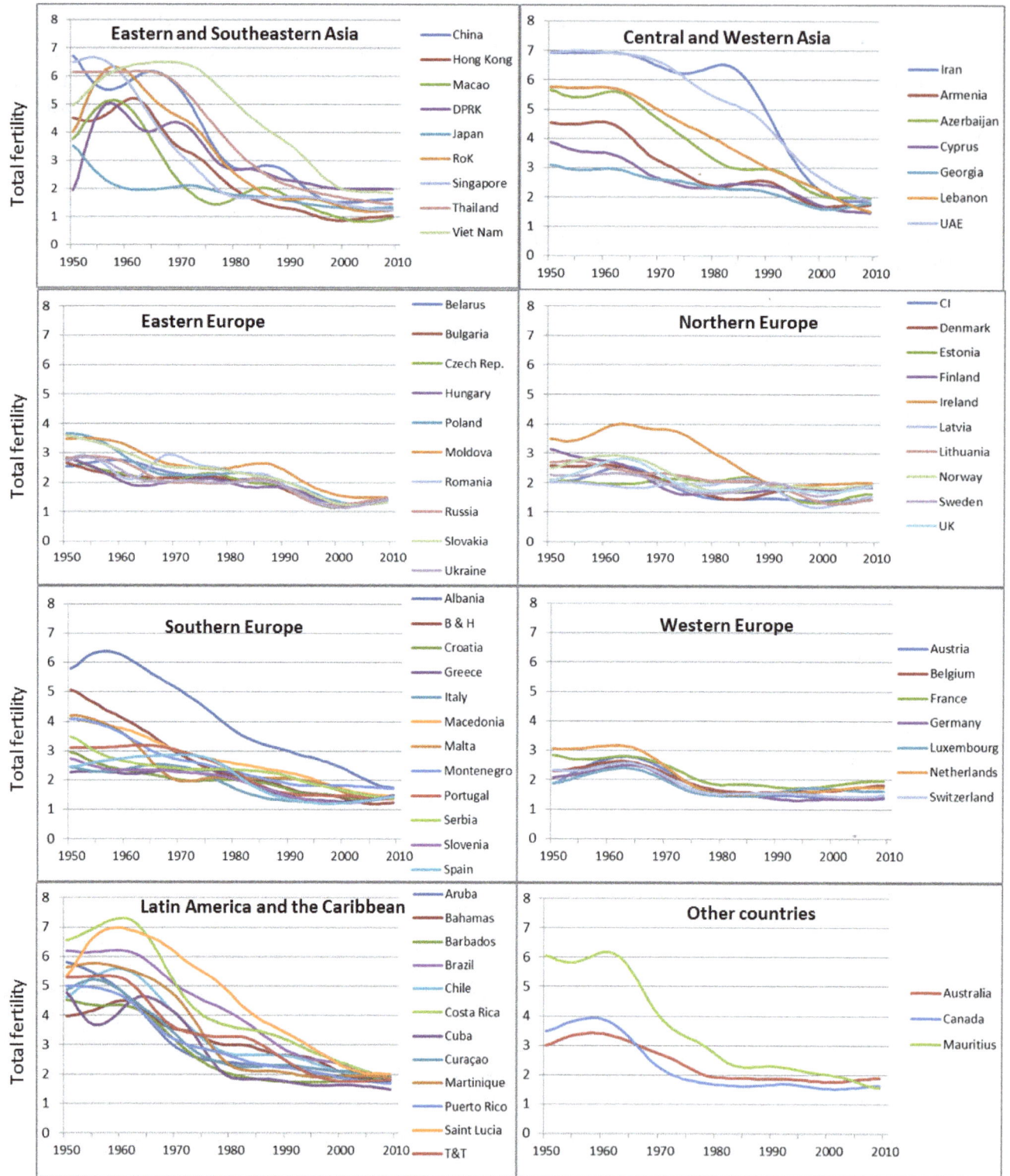

Source: United Nations (2013a).

NOTES: B&H refers to Bosnia and Herzegovina, CI refers to Channel Islands, Czech Rep. refers to Czech Republic, DPRK refers to Democratic People's Republic of Korea, RoK refers to Republic of Korea, T&T refers to Trinidad and Tobago, UAE refers to United Arab Emirates, and UK refers to United Kingdom.

B. FERTILITY DECLINE AT YOUNG AND OLD AGES

1. *Adolescent fertility*

Though all countries in this study have below-replacement fertility, many still have a relatively high proportion of births to adolescent mothers. Low-fertility countries in Latin America and the Caribbean have relatively high adolescent birth rates (ABR) in 2005-2010 (figure I.3), ranging from 22 births per 1,000 women aged 15-19 in Martinique to 76 births per 1,000 women aged 15-19 in Brazil. The decline in adolescent fertility in low-fertility countries in Latin America and the Caribbean since 1990-1995 has been more modest than in low-fertility countries in other regions that also had high adolescent fertility in 1990-1995, such as Eastern Europe and Central and Western Asia. Moreover, adolescent fertility in Latin America and the Caribbean is defined by very high differentials by socio-economic and education group (Cavenaghi, 2013). In 8 of 12 countries in Latin America and the Caribbean, the ABR declined by less than one third between 1990-1995 and 2005-2010, and between one third and a half in the remainder of the countries (an exception is the Bahamas, where the ABR declined by more than half). In Brazil, for example, the ABR declined from 84 births per 1,000 women aged 15-19 in 1990-1995 to 76 in 2005-2010 (a decline of less than 10 per cent). Armenia had a similar adolescent birth rate to Brazil in 1990-1995 of 80 births per 1,000 women aged 15-19, but by 2005-2010 this had declined by about 65 per cent to 28 births per 1,000 women aged 15-19.

Central and Western Asia and Eastern Europe have relatively high adolescent birth rates. Eastern Europe has higher adolescent birth rates than other sub-regions of Europe, although there have been sharp declines in many countries since 1990-1995. In Northern Europe, the countries from the former Soviet Union (Estonia, Latvia and Lithuania) and Ireland and United Kingdom have relatively high adolescent birth rates, although Estonia, Latvia and Lithuania have experienced declines of more than half since 1990-1995.

Eastern and South-Eastern Asia stand out as regions with very low adolescent fertility, both in 1990-1995 and 2005-2010 with the notable exceptions of Thailand and Viet Nam where the ABR in 2005-2010 was 41 and 32, respectively. Western Europe also stands out as a region with particularly low adolescent birth rates (less than 11 births per 1,000 women aged 15-19). Other countries in Northern Europe all had very low adolescent birth rates of 9 births or below per 1,000 women aged 15-19.

The bubble sizes in figure I.3 represent the proportion of the total fertility attributed to births to adolescents aged 15-19 years, which is high in low-fertility countries in Latin America and the Caribbean compared to other regions. In 2005-2010, 10 of 18 low-fertility countries where the proportion of period total fertility attributable to adolescent fertility is 10 per cent or more are in Latin America and the Caribbean. In four of these countries (Brazil, Chile, Costa Rica and Saint Lucia), the ABR increased between 1990-1995 and 2005-2010. Thailand, in South-Eastern Asia and Azerbaijan, in Western Asia, are the other low-fertility countries where the ABR constitutes 10 per cent or more of total fertility and where the ABR increased. Given that reducing childbearing among adolescents is a concern of many Governments, reductions in adolescent childbearing will likely be associated with further reductions in overall fertility levels.

**Figure I.3. Adolescent birth rate (ABR) in 1990-1995 and 2005-2010
and adolescent birth rate as a percentage of total fertility (TF) in 2005-2010, low-fertility countries**

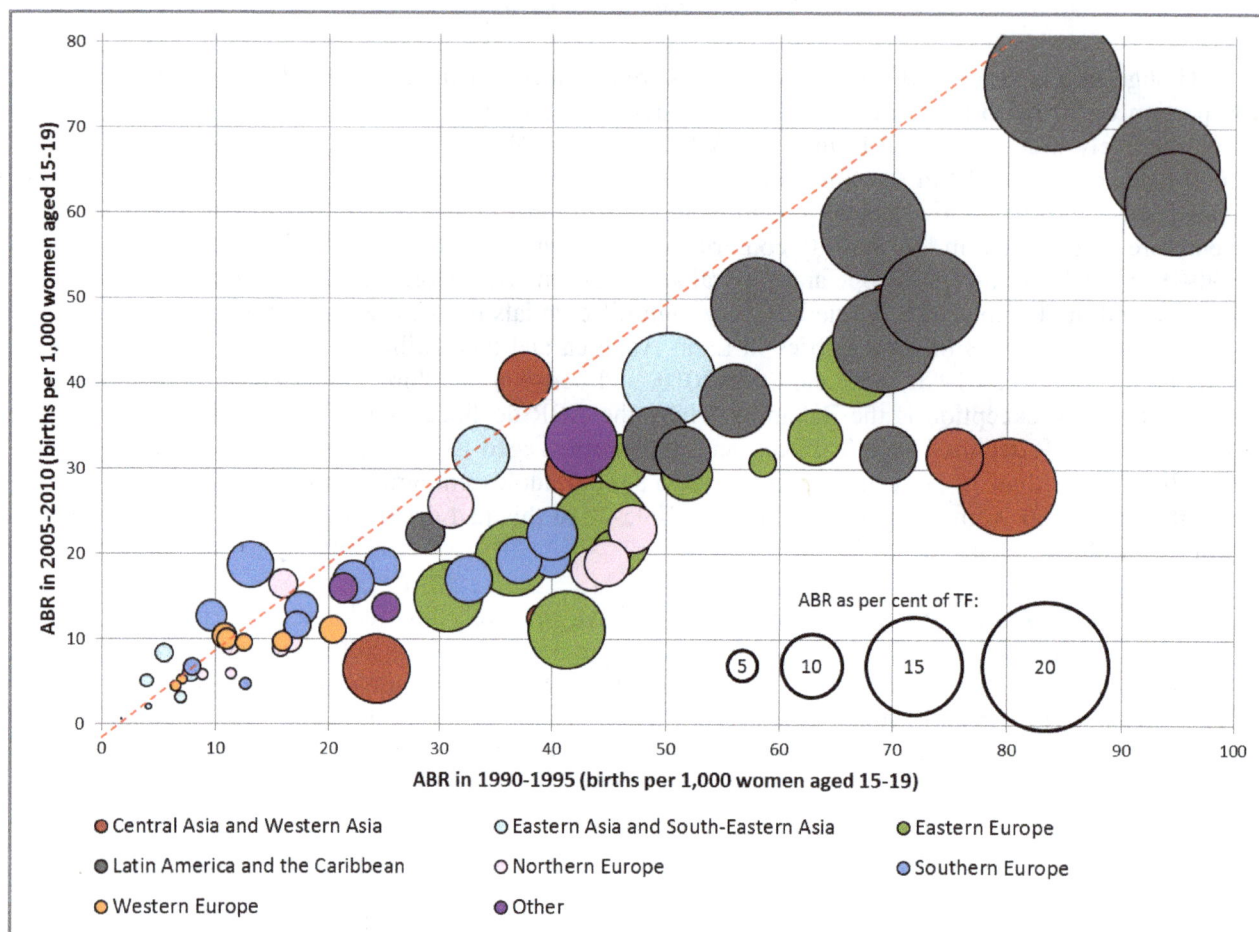

Source: United Nations (2013a).
NOTE: The bubble size represents the proportion of the total fertility attributed to births to adolescents aged 15-19 years.

2. Postponement of childbearing

The postponement of the start of childbearing to older ages is increasingly a feature of low-fertility countries. Nearly all low-fertility countries with available data have had an increase in the mean age at first birth since the 1994 ICPD (figure I.4). There were no countries with a mean age at first birth of 30 years or older at the time of the ICPD, and yet the most recent data points available show that four low-fertility countries had a mean age at first birth of 30 years or older. Countries in Northern Europe, Western Europe, Eastern Asia and South-Eastern Asia retained their pattern over time of having among the oldest ages at first birth. In many countries in Eastern Europe and Southern Europe, the age at first birth has significantly increased. In some of these countries, the pace of increase since circa 1994 was three years or more per decade. In contrast, the age at first birth in low-fertility countries in Central Asia and Western Asia has remained young (the exception is Cyprus).

Figure I.4. Mean age at first birth, around 1994 and latest point available, low-fertility countries

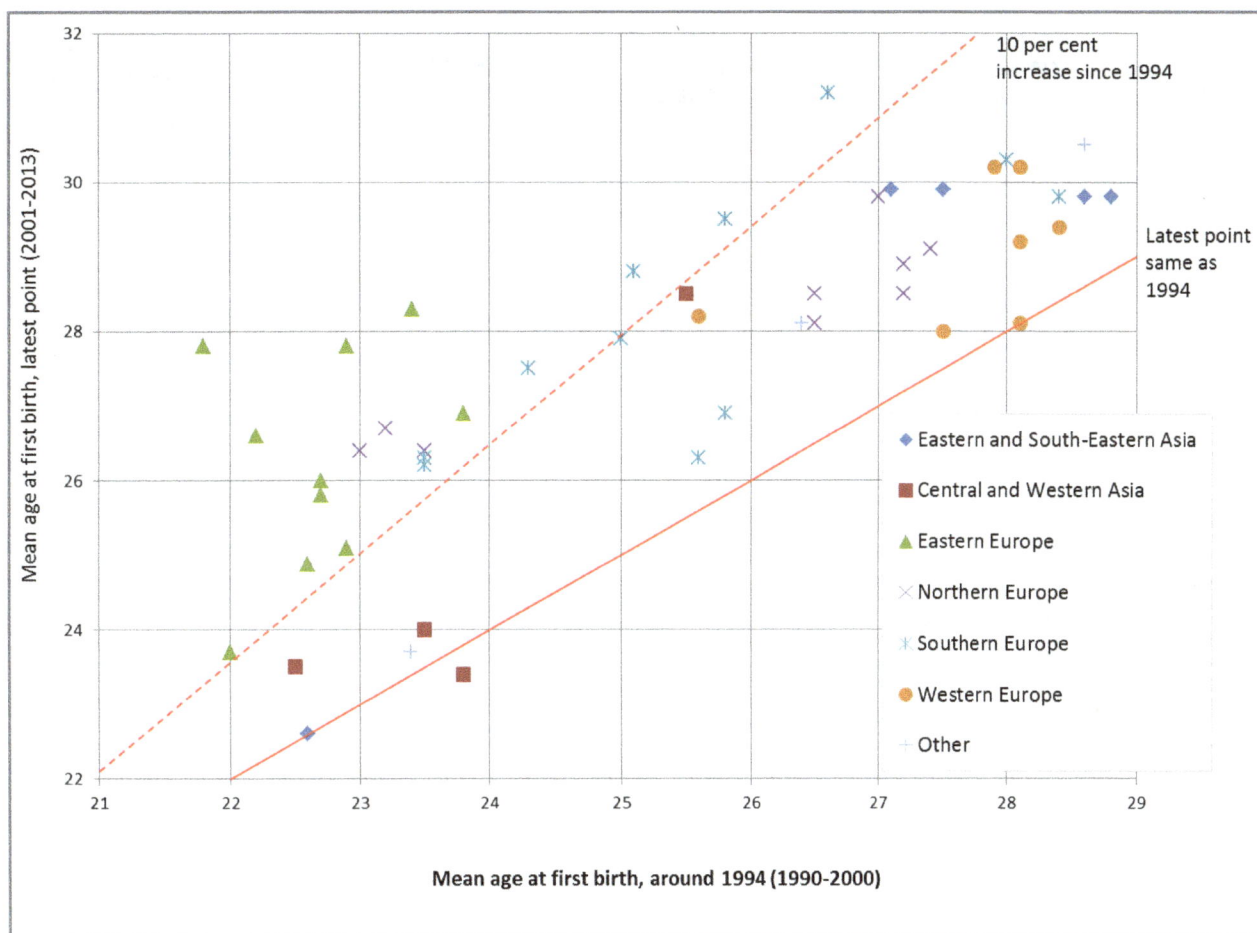

Source: National sources. See annex table 2 for detailed sources.

3. *Fertility of older women*

Increasingly, in low-fertility countries, women are giving birth at older ages (figure I.5). Adverse perinatal and maternal outcomes, including low birth weight, preterm delivery, birth defects and perinatal mortality are generally higher for older women, as well as issues around infertility due to the postponement of childbearing.

In 45 of the 70 low-fertility countries, there has been an increase in the fertility rate among 40-44 years old women, primarily due to the postponement of births at younger ages. The largest increase has tended to be in countries in Northern Europe, Southern Europe and Western Europe. The fertility rate of women aged 40-44 years increased by twofold or more since 1990-1995 in 11 low-fertility countries in Europe (Belgium, Czech Republic, Denmark, Estonia, Germany, Greece, Italy, Luxembourg, Romania, Slovenia and Switzerland) and in Australia, Barbados and Japan.

Figure I.5. Number of births per 1,000 women aged 40-44, 1990-1995 and 2005-2010, low-fertility countries

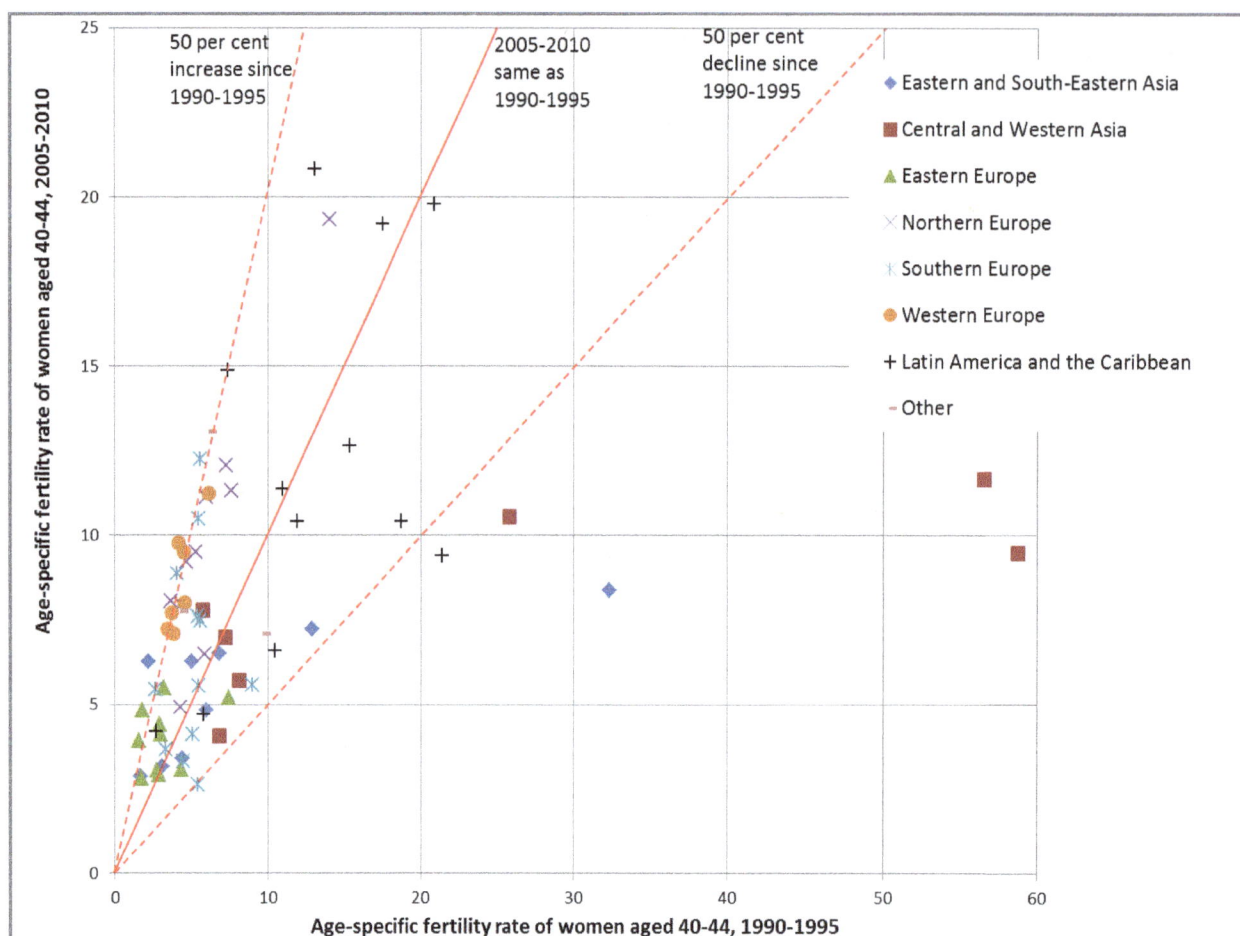

Source: United Nations (2013a).

In countries that had more recent fertility transitions, predominantly in Central Asia, Western Asia, and Latin America and the Caribbean, there have been sharp decreases in the fertility rate of women aged 40-44 years. Brazil, Costa Rica, Iran, Lebanon, United Arab Emirates and Viet Nam stand out as having had particularly large declines in the fertility rate of older women. In Iran, the number of births per 1,000 women aged 40-44 years decreased from 57 in 1990-1995 to 12 in 2005-2010 and in the United Arab Emirates, the decline was from 59 to 10 births per 1,000 women aged 40-44 years.

In most low-fertility countries, the proportion of total fertility attributable to births among women aged 40-44 years has increased (figure I.6), and this is particularly the case in Europe where most low-fertility countries experienced increases in fertility at older ages from relatively low levels in 1990-1995. In each of the 45 low-fertility countries where the fertility rate of women aged 40-44 years increased, the proportion of total fertility attributable to women in this age group increased. Cyprus and Singapore are the only countries where the proportion of total fertility attributable to women aged 40-44 years increased despite a decline in the fertility rate of women in this age group. The largest absolute increase (2 to 3 per cent) occurred in Australia, Bahamas, Barbados, Greece, Italy, Japan, Luxembourg, Spain and Switzerland. In countries that had a sharp decline in the fertility rate of women aged 40-44 years, the proportion of total fertility attributable to women in this age group also decreased. These countries include Brazil, Costa Rica, Iran, Lebanon, Thailand, United Arab Emirates and Viet Nam. In 2005-2010, the proportion of total fertility attributable to the fertility of women aged 40-44 years ranges from 1 to 3 per cent in 28 low-fertility countries. Twenty-one of these countries are in Europe; the other countries are Australia, Bahamas, Barbados, Canada, Hong Kong SAR of China, Japan and Saint Lucia.

Figure I.6. Proportion of total fertility attributable to births to women aged 40-44, 1990-1995 and 2005-2010, low-fertility countries

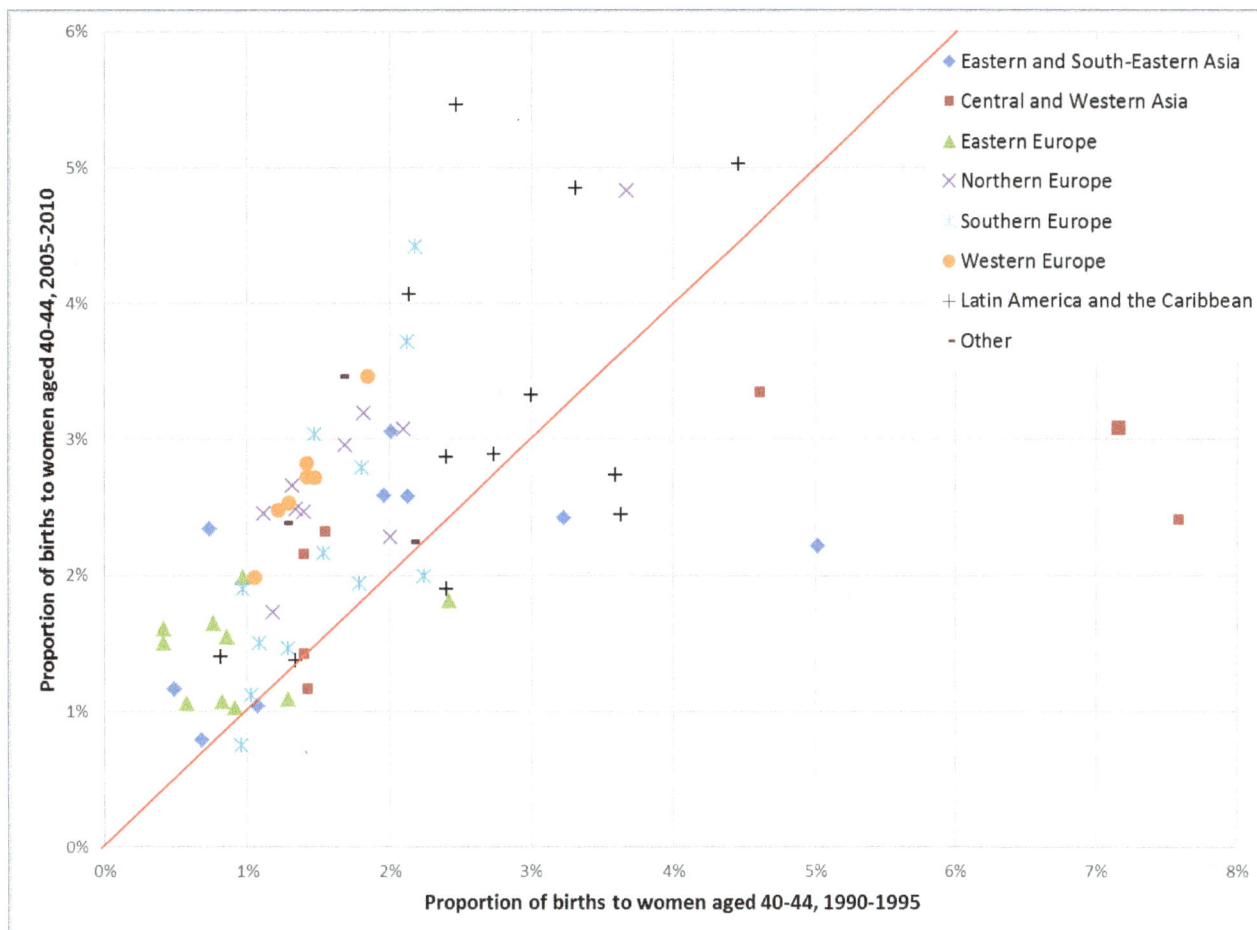

Source: United Nations (2013a).

4. *Overall age pattern of fertility*

The overall distribution of age-specific fertility rates among low-fertility countries further illustrates the wide variation in age patterns of childbearing even when total fertility levels are similar (figure I.7). The younger childbearing pattern in many countries in Eastern Europe and Latin America and the Caribbean and the later childbearing pattern in many countries in Northern Europe and Western Europe is clear. In Latin America and the Caribbean, fertility is more concentrated at ages below 30 years, with most countries reflecting high levels of adolescent fertility and peak fertility in the age group 20-24 years. Brazil illustrates this pattern. Childbearing in Eastern Europe also tends to be concentrated among women in their twenties.

Figure I.7. Age-specific fertility rates among low-fertility countries by region, 2005-2010

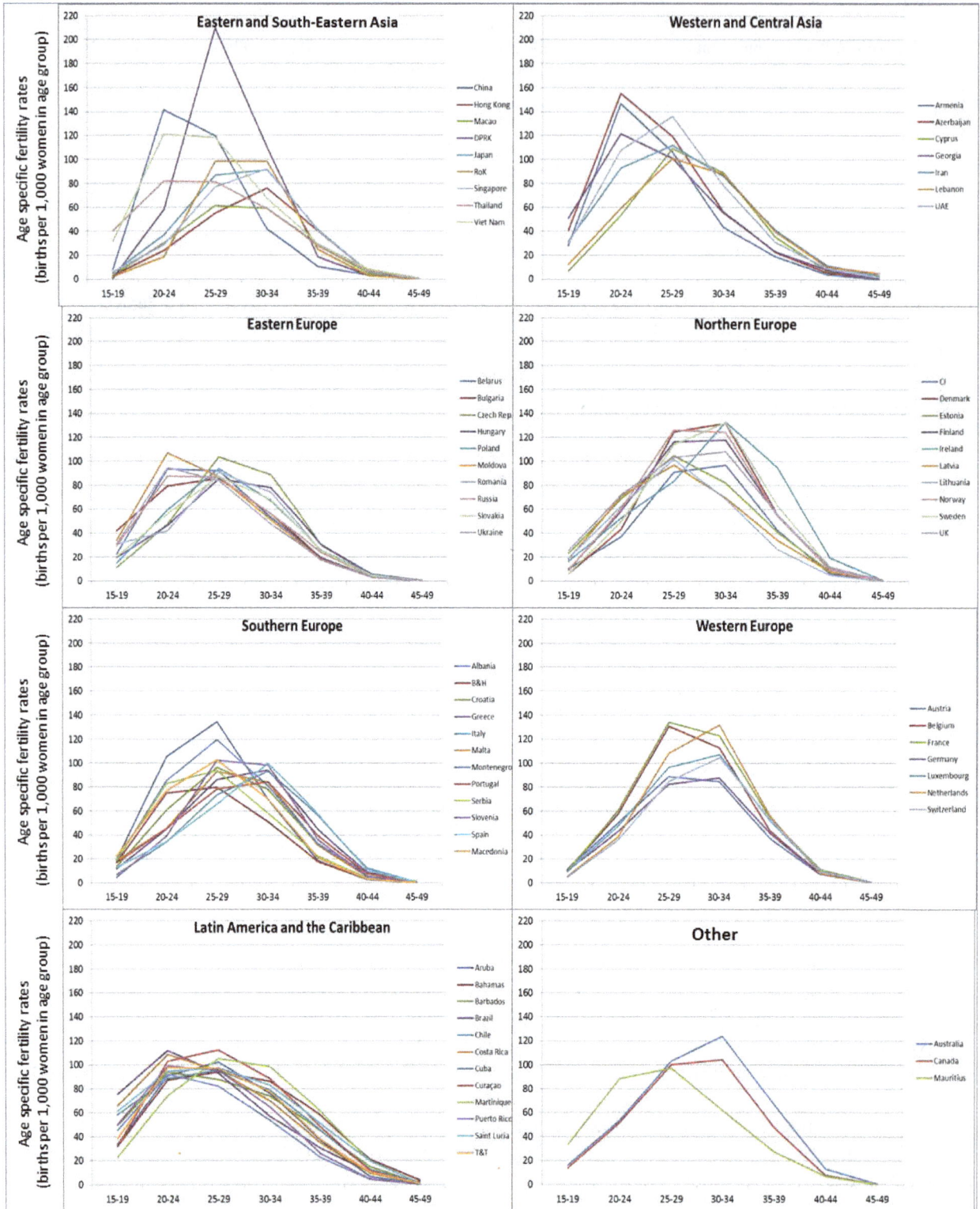

Source: United Nations (2013a).

All countries in Northern Europe, Southern Europe and Western Europe have peak childbearing in the 25-29 or 30-34 years age groups. Albania and Montenegro stand out as having childbearing concentrated in younger age groups and Ireland has relatively high levels of childbearing at older ages. Most countries in Central Asia and Western Asia tend to have a relatively early peak in fertility, and all countries have peak fertility between the ages of 20 and 29 years. In Eastern Asia and South-Eastern Asia there is wide variation among countries in the age pattern of childbearing. Some countries, such as China and Viet Nam, show a peak level of fertility in the 20-24 years age group, while Hong Kong SAR of China, Japan and Singapore all have a later peak in fertility in the 30-34 years age group.

C. COMPLETED FERTILITY AND CHILDLESSNESS

While the age-specific period fertility rates provide a picture of fertility at a particular point in time, completed fertility is a function of historical fertility rates experienced by women as they passed through their childbearing years. Often the period fertility rates can decline to levels that are much lower than completed fertility by cohort because the period rates are sensitive to the timing of childbearing and a shift to childbearing at older ages (a "tempo" effect). In other words, if women decide to postpone childbearing to older ages, the years in which the postponement occurs will record fewer births and a lower period measure of total fertility.

The distribution of the number of children born to women who have completed or are approaching the end of their childbearing years also provides information on the different routes by which countries have reached low fertility. Completed family size, measured here by the number of children ever born to women aged 40-44 years, reflects past fertility behaviour and, as such, may differ from period total fertility, especially where fertility decline has been rapid.

In some countries, a relatively high proportion of women remain childless but the women who do have children tend to have large families. In other countries, childlessness is less common but women who have children tend to have smaller families of one or two children. For the purposes of this report, childlessness is defined as women who have not had a live birth, regardless of whether women are intentionally childless or not.

Most low-fertility countries experienced an increase in childlessness among women aged 40-44 years since the 1994 ICPD (points above the solid diagonal line in figure I.8). Childlessness exceeded 20 per cent of women aged 40-44 years for the most recent period in 5 of the 45 low-fertility countries with data for both periods, while no country had this level of childlessness around 1994. The level of childlessness among older women more than doubled between 1994 and the latest period in Austria, Japan, Spain and Thailand. The highest rates of childlessness are currently in European and Eastern Asian low-fertility countries (figure I.9), with Singapore having the highest level of childlessness (23 per cent of women aged 40-44 years).

Yet many low-fertility countries still have low levels of childlessness among women aged 40-44 years, especially countries with more recent fertility transitions. Levels of childlessness tend to be lower in countries in Eastern Europe, Central Asia, Western Asia and some countries in Southern Europe, with even a decrease in childlessness in some of these countries. For example, Lebanon, Mauritius and Portugal all have levels of childlessness among women aged 40-44 years of below 5 per cent.

Low-fertility countries also vary in the proportion of older women who have completed family sizes of three or more children, even in countries with similar levels of period total fertility. As with the lower levels of childlessness, countries with the highest percentage of women aged 40-44 years with three or more children ever born also tend to be countries that made a more recent transition to below-replacement fertility (figure I.9). However, even in countries that had low fertility for decades, there is still much variation in family size. In many countries, especially in Eastern Europe, a complete family size of three or more children is relatively rare as is childlessness, with most women having one or two children. In contrast, in other countries, predominantly in Northern Europe and Western Europe, both childlessness and family sizes of three or more children are more common.

Figure I.8. Percentage of women aged 40-44 who are childless, around 1994 and latest point available, low-fertility countries

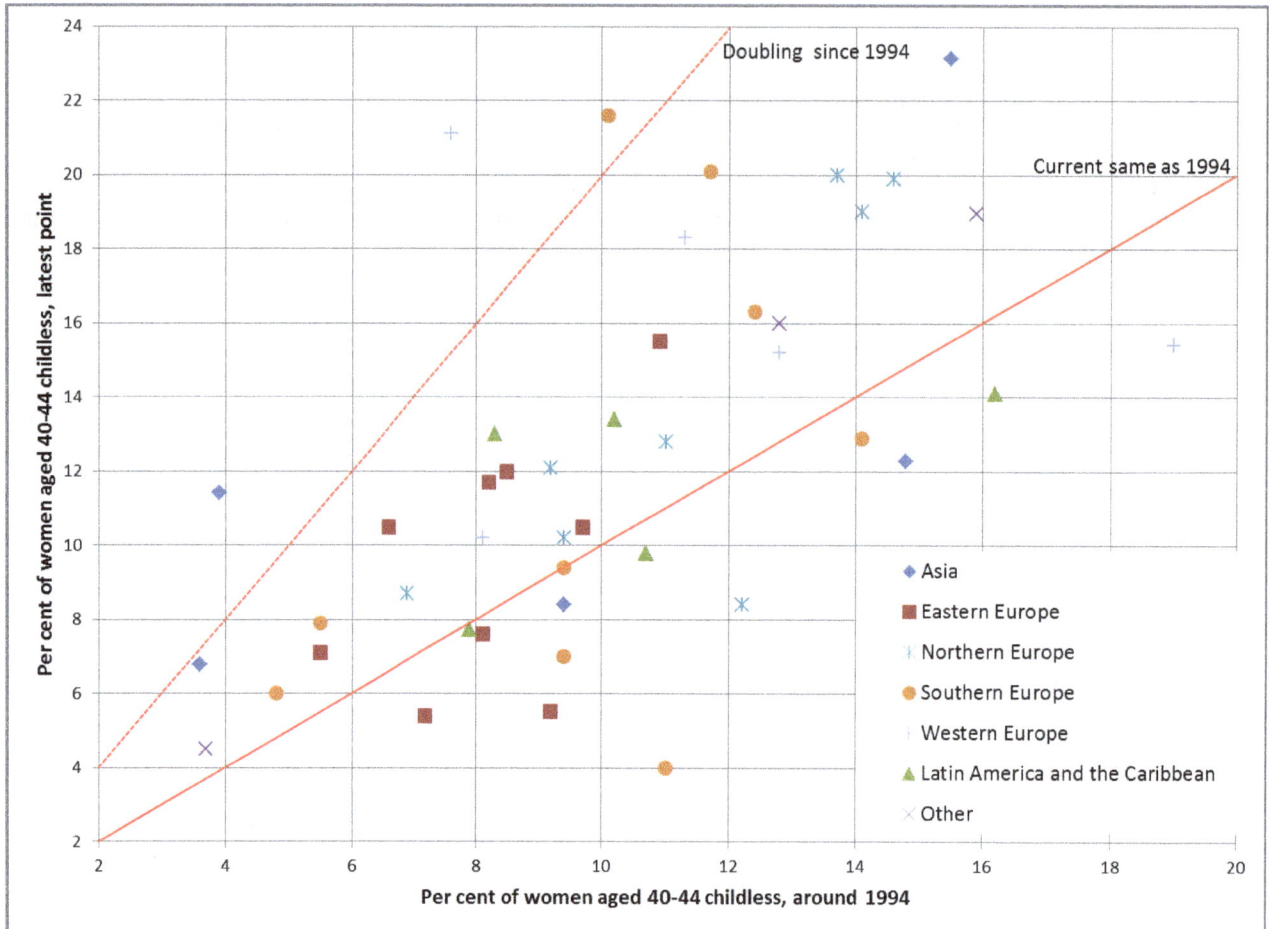

Source: National Sources. See annex table 3 for detailed sources.

Figure I.9. Percentage of women aged 40-44 who are childless or with three or more children, latest point available, low-fertility countries

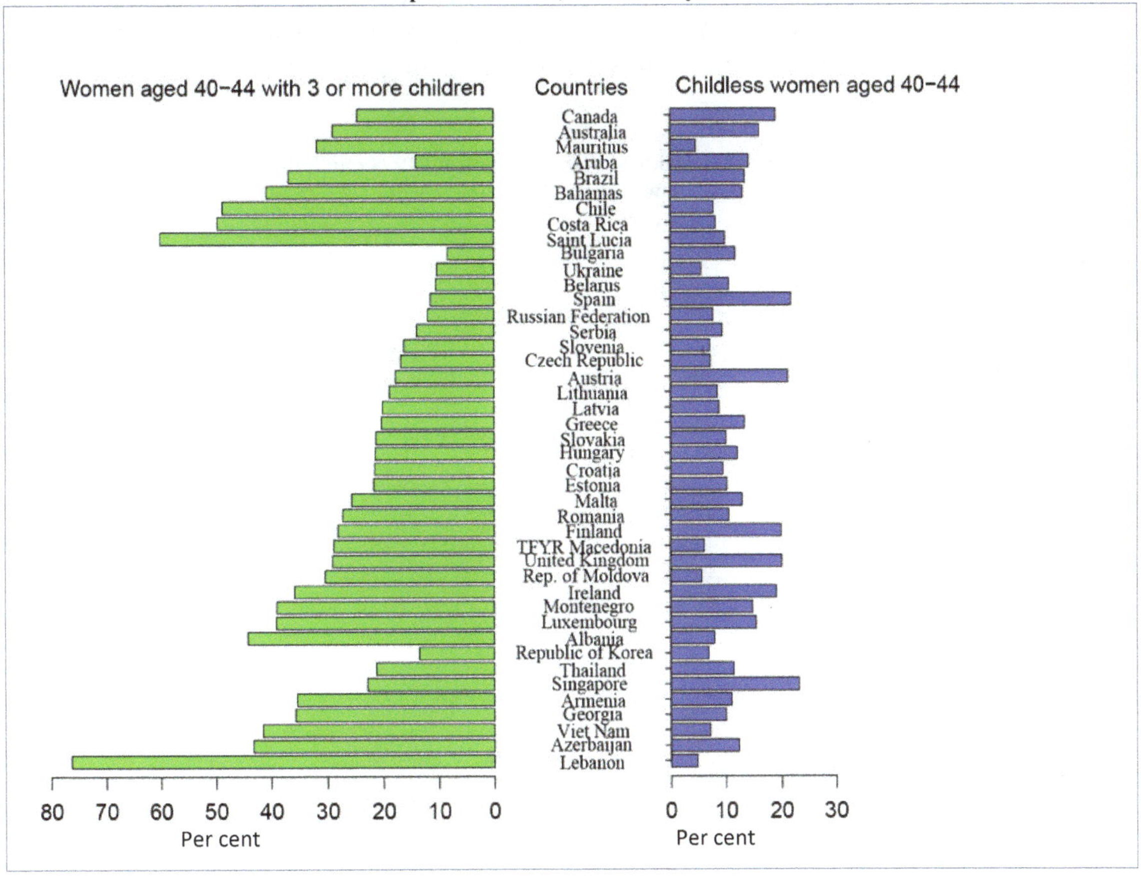
Women aged 40−44 with 3 or more children
Countries
Childless women aged 40−44
Canada
Australia
Mauritius
Aruba
Brazil
Bahamas
Chile
Costa Rica
Saint Lucia
Bulgaria
Ukraine
Belarus
Spain
Russian Federation
Serbia
Slovenia
Czech Republic
Austria
Lithuania
Latvia
Greece
Slovakia
Hungary
Croatia
Estonia
Malta
Romania
Finland
TFYR Macedonia
United Kingdom
Rep. of Moldova
Ireland
Montenegro
Luxembourg
Albania
Republic of Korea
Thailand
Singapore
Armenia
Georgia
Viet Nam
Azerbaijan
Lebanon
80 70 60 50 40 30 20 10 0
Per cent
0 10 20 30
Per cent

Source: National Sources. See annex table 3 for detailed sources.

D. CHILDBEARING AND MARRIAGE

Marriage patterns, including the timing of marriage and the proportion of women and men who have ever been married, have an influence on fertility levels and the timing of births. The analysis of childbearing and marriage is complex because the nature of unions in which childbearing occurs goes beyond formal marriage to include consensual unions and other types of unions. Moreover, comparable data on union status across countries and over time are limited. Despite these analytical challenges, several recent trends in childbearing and union formation characterize low-fertility countries.

1. *Childbearing outside of marriage*

One of the most profound changes in fertility is the rise in childbearing outside of marriage. There is stark variation by region in patterns of childbearing outside of marriage, and while these births may not occur within a formal marriage, they may still be within a cohabiting union. Among 49 low-fertility countries with data available for both around 1994 and the latest period, there has been a clear increase in the proportion of births outside of marriage. At least 40 per cent of births occurred outside of marriage in 21 countries in the latest period (figure I.10), an increase from only 9 countries around 1994. The majority of these countries are in Northern Europe and Latin America and the Caribbean, where women have traditionally had high levels of births outside of formal marriage. Extra-marital childbearing in many countries of these regions was already common around 1994, including in Estonia, Latvia, and Lithuania, where extra-marital births increased rapidly following the disintegration of the Soviet Union in 1991.

In contrast, extra-marital births were less common in countries in Western Europe around 1994, at levels of less than 20 per cent in five of the seven countries with data. Rapid increases have since occurred in these countries (figure I.10). France has the highest proportion of extra-marital births in Western Europe and is 1 of the 12 low-fertility countries where 50 per cent or more of births occur outside of marriage.

Figure I.10. Percentage of births outside of marriage, around 1994 and latest point available, low-fertility countries

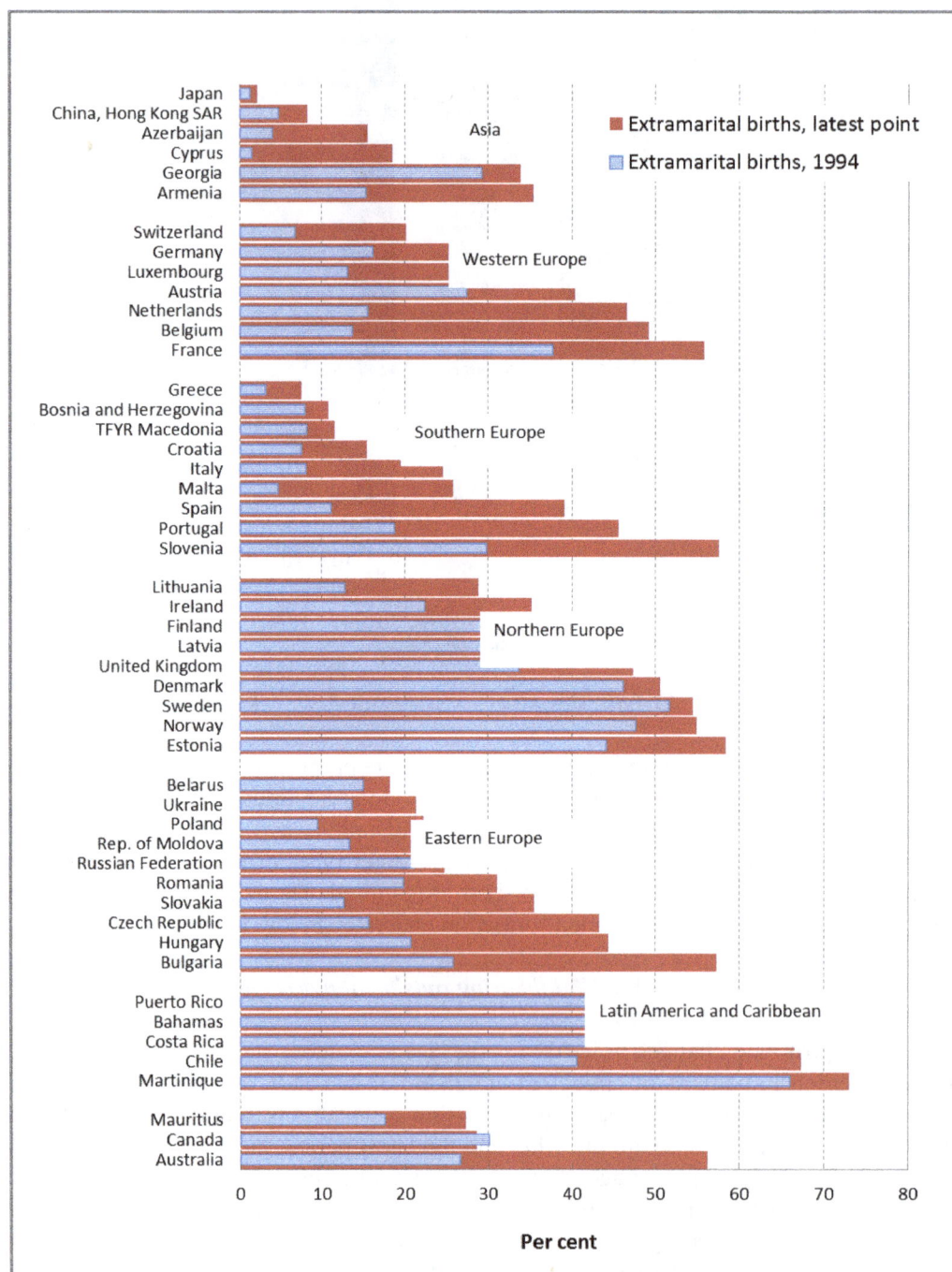

Source: National sources. See annex table 4 for detailed sources.

The level of childbearing outside of marriage among most countries in Eastern Europe and Southern Europe is lower compared to Northern Europe and Western Europe. However, substantial increases have occurred since 1994 in the majority of countries of these regions. Childbearing outside of marriage is relatively uncommon among the low-fertility countries in Asia, though the percentage of extra-marital births has more than doubled in all low-fertility countries in this region, except Georgia and Japan.

2. *Increase in mean age at marriage*

A higher average age at which men and women marry is associated with the postponement of childbearing and the proportion of men and women who ultimately remain unmarried, although, as has been shown already, the link between childbearing and marriage is increasingly weakening.

In nearly all 59 low-fertility countries with trend data, there has been an increase in the age at first marriage (figure I.11).[3] Around 1994, the mean age at first marriage for women was above 30 years in only two countries, France and Sweden. For the most recent year, 16 of the 59 low-fertility countries now have a mean age at first marriage among women in excess of 30 years, all of them in Europe except Hong Kong SAR of China. In the Czech Republic and Latvia, for example, the mean age at first marriage for women has risen by more than seven years from around 1994 to the most recent period.

3. *Changes in the proportion of women who have never married*

Change in the proportion of women who have never married also accounts for part of the trend in childbearing in low-fertility countries. In some countries, especially in Latin America and the Caribbean, consensual unions have effectively replaced marriage. This is also increasingly the case in Northern Europe and Western Europe, where never-married women often live in consensual unions.

---

[3] Estimates of the average age at first marriage are based on the singulate mean age at marriage, a measure of the average length of single life expressed in years among those who marry before age 50 years and calculated from cross-sectional census or survey data on the proportions of never-married men and women at each age between 15 and 54 years. Data are available for 59 of the 70 low-fertility countries.

Figure I.11. Female mean age at first marriage, around 1994 and latest point available, low-fertility countries

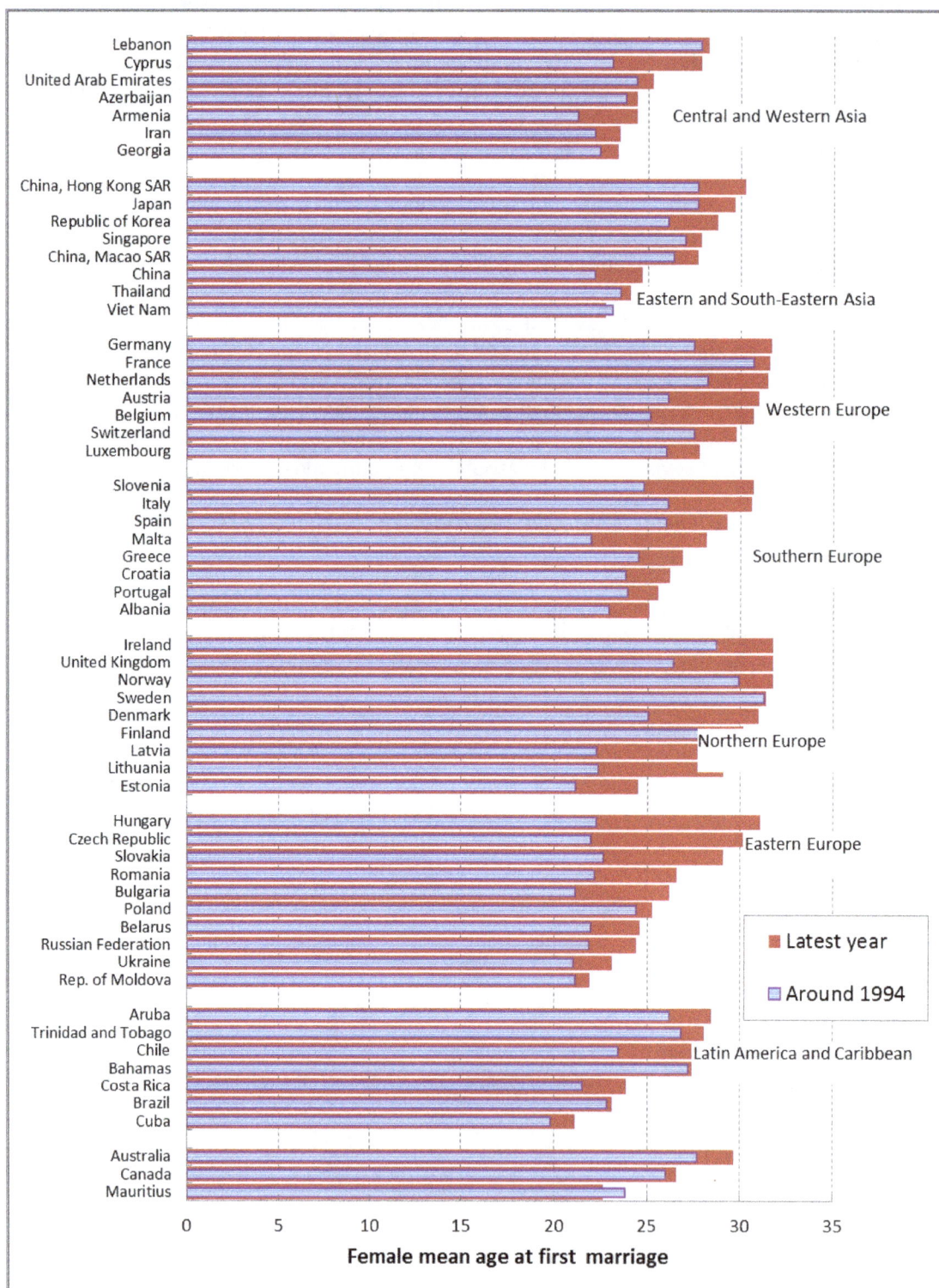

Source: United Nations (2013b).

    World Fertility Report 2013: Fertility at the Extremes

Figure I.12. Percentage of women aged 40-44 who never married, around 1994 and latest point available, low-fertility countries

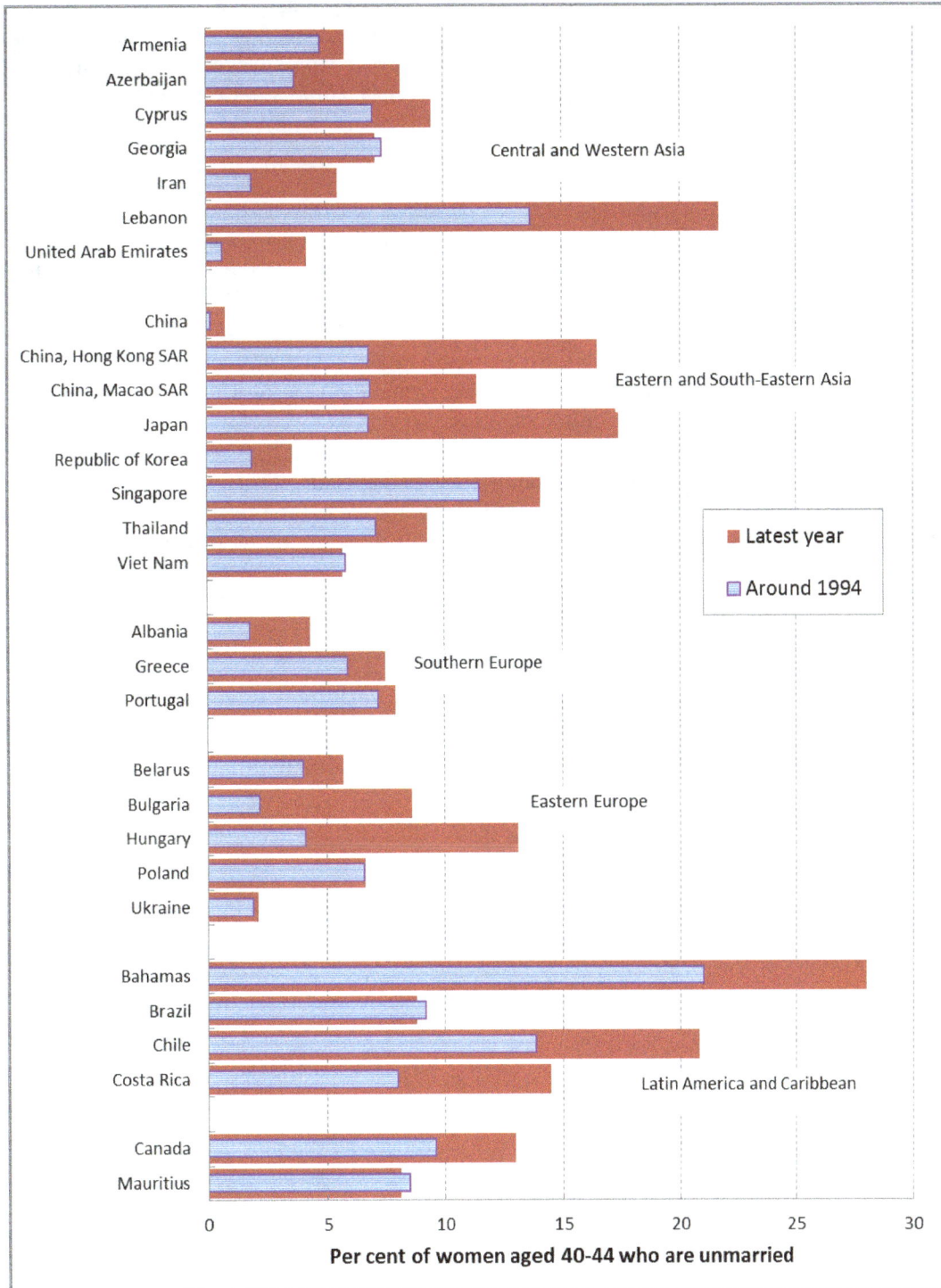

Per cent of women aged 40-44 who are unmarried

Legend:
- ■ Latest year
- ☐ Around 1994

Regional groupings shown: Central and Western Asia; Eastern and South-Eastern Asia; Southern Europe; Eastern Europe; Latin America and Caribbean

Source: United Nations 2013b.

NOTES: The figures only include countries where consensual unions were reported as a separate category for marital status in data collection for both periods. The exceptions are Albania and Poland where data showed that consensual unions are below 4 per cent or in countries in Asia where consensual unions are assumed to be rare.

The proportion of women aged 40-44 years who have never married increased since around 1994 in most low-fertility countries, although there is a wide range in levels (figure I.12). The increase has been particularly large in countries in Eastern Asia. Where childbearing outside of marriage is uncommon, as in most parts of Asia, this trend means that the postponement or rejection of marriage is an important determinant of fertility levels. The proportion of never-married women aged 40-44 years has reached levels of more than 20 per cent in countries such as the Bahamas, Chile and Lebanon.

E. FERTILITY PROJECTIONS

Much debate exists regarding future fertility levels in low-fertility countries (Lutz and others, 2014; United Nations, 2013a). The projections described here assume a slight increase in fertility over time for countries that have already reached around or below replacement-level fertility and where the pace of fertility decline has decreased to zero. This pattern of a slight increase in fertility following declines to low levels is one that has been experienced in at least 25 low-fertility countries or areas, 16 of which are in Northern Europe or Western Europe (United Nations, 2014b). The projection model also allows for country-specific variability in the pace of fertility recovery and the long-term fertility level reached based on each country's historical experience (United Nations, 2014b).

Most low-fertility countries, especially countries with very low fertility (below 1.6 children per woman in 2005-2010), are projected to experience slight increases in total fertility to 2030-2035 under the medium fertility variant, although fertility rates will still be well below replacement level (figure I.13).

Figure I.13. Total fertility (TF) for countries by major area, estimates for 2005-2010 and projections for 2030-2035, low-fertility countries

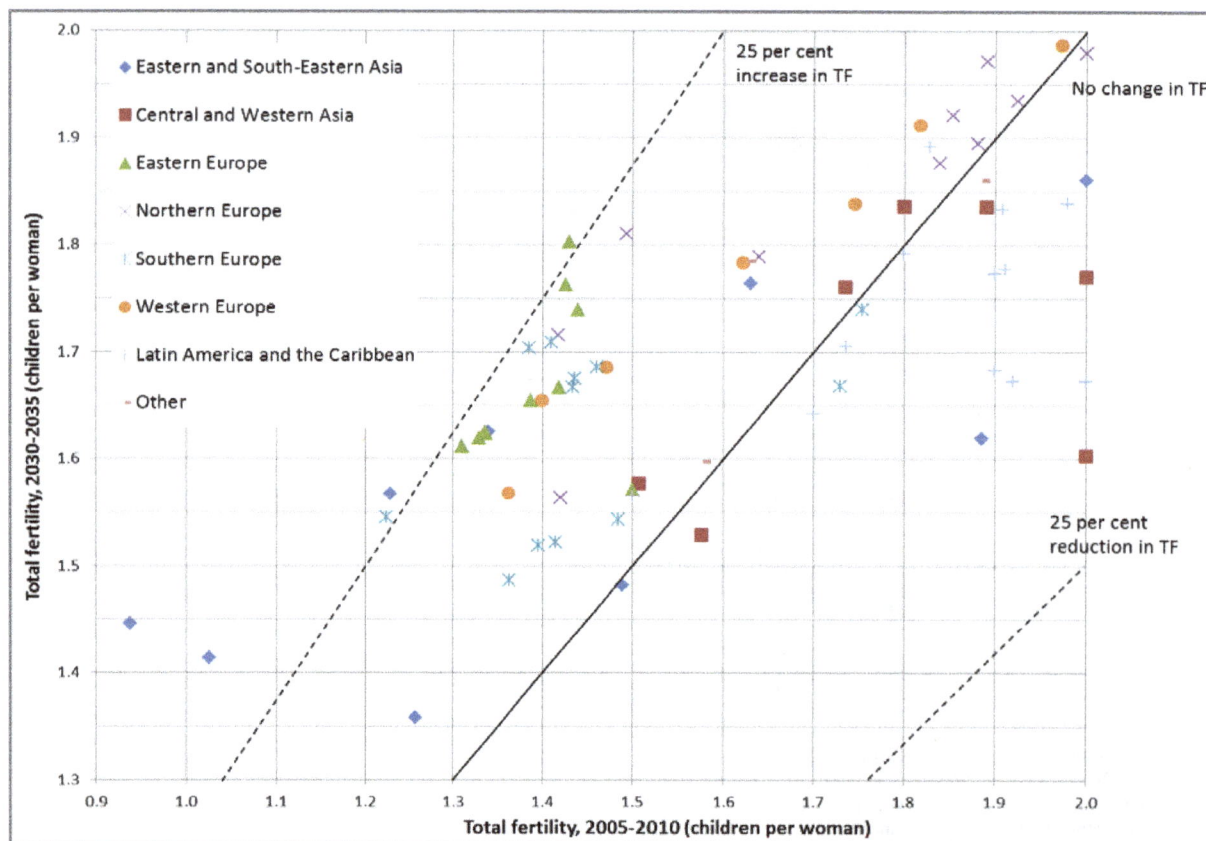

Source: United Nations (2013a).

Altogether, the number of low-fertility countries or areas with total fertility below 1.6 children per woman is projected to decrease from 34 countries in 2005-2010 to 10 countries in 2030-2035. Many low-fertility countries outside of Europe, predominantly those with more recent fertility transitions and higher total fertility, are projected to have a continued fertility decline to 2030-2035.

F. CONSEQUENCES OF LOW FERTILITY

At the time of the 1994 ICPD, low fertility was mainly a characteristic of high-income countries, especially in Europe. Since that time, low fertility has also become a feature of middle-income countries, which have more limited resources to address many of the consequences of low fertility compared to high-income countries. Moreover, many of these middle-income countries have experienced far more rapid transitions to low fertility levels than was historically the case and thus these countries have had less time to adapt to the resulting macro-level changes.

The most obvious long-term consequence of sustained low fertility is population ageing. In countries where the fertility transition has been rapid and recent, the population is often still relatively youthful due to large cohorts of people of working age, compared with countries with more established fertility transitions. Consequently, countries with more recent fertility transitions have had a smaller increase in the old-age dependency ratio (the ratio of the population aged 70 years or over to the population aged 20 to 69 years) between 1995 and 2015 compared with countries that have had low fertility levels for a long period (figure I.14).

The increase in the old-age dependency ratio between 2015 and 2035 is projected to be substantial for all low-fertility countries, especially countries in regions apart from Europe, where the old-age dependency ratio is projected to double. This increase in the older population compared to the working-age population will present a serious challenge to these countries, especially since many of them are middle-income countries or countries where the care of older persons has traditionally been a family responsibility (Guo, 2012; Stephen, 2012).

Another consequence of low fertility is the increased reliance by countries on positive net in-migration to meet labour market needs. Although international migration is not a long-term structural remedy for population ageing, it can help mitigate the short-term effects of an ageing population. Migration can increase the working-age population, and migrant women often tend to be of reproductive age and to have, at least initially, higher fertility rates (Wilson and others, 2013). High levels of migration to a country, while associated with lower levels of fertility, is not perfectly correlated with fertility levels. In other words, in-migration may be low where fertility is also low (such as Ukraine) or, conversely, there may be high levels of in-migration where fertility is relatively high (such as France). Furthermore, migration as a mitigation strategy for low fertility may not be appropriate for all low-fertility countries, especially given that low fertility is occurring at ever-lower levels of development and the political sensitivities around migration in some countries. For example, countries in Eastern and South-Eastern Europe, which have struggling economies, have both low levels of fertility and net out-migration, leading to even more significant population decline (Sobotka, 2013; Wilson and others, 2013). Many low-fertility countries in Asia have far lower migration levels than European countries (Abbassi and Gubhaju, 2014).

In the absence of migration, population size will begin to decrease if fertility levels remain stable at a below-replacement level. In 1990-1995, there were 12 countries with a negative rate of natural increase (i.e., deaths outnumbered births), all of which were in Europe (the exception was Rwanda due to the genocide in 1994). By 2010-2015, 17 countries are projected to have a negative rate of natural increase, all of which are in Europe, except Japan. By 2030-2035, 40 countries are projected to have a negative rate of natural increase, including 9 countries in regions other than Europe.

Figure I.14. Old-age dependency ratio, 1995 to 2035, low-fertility countries

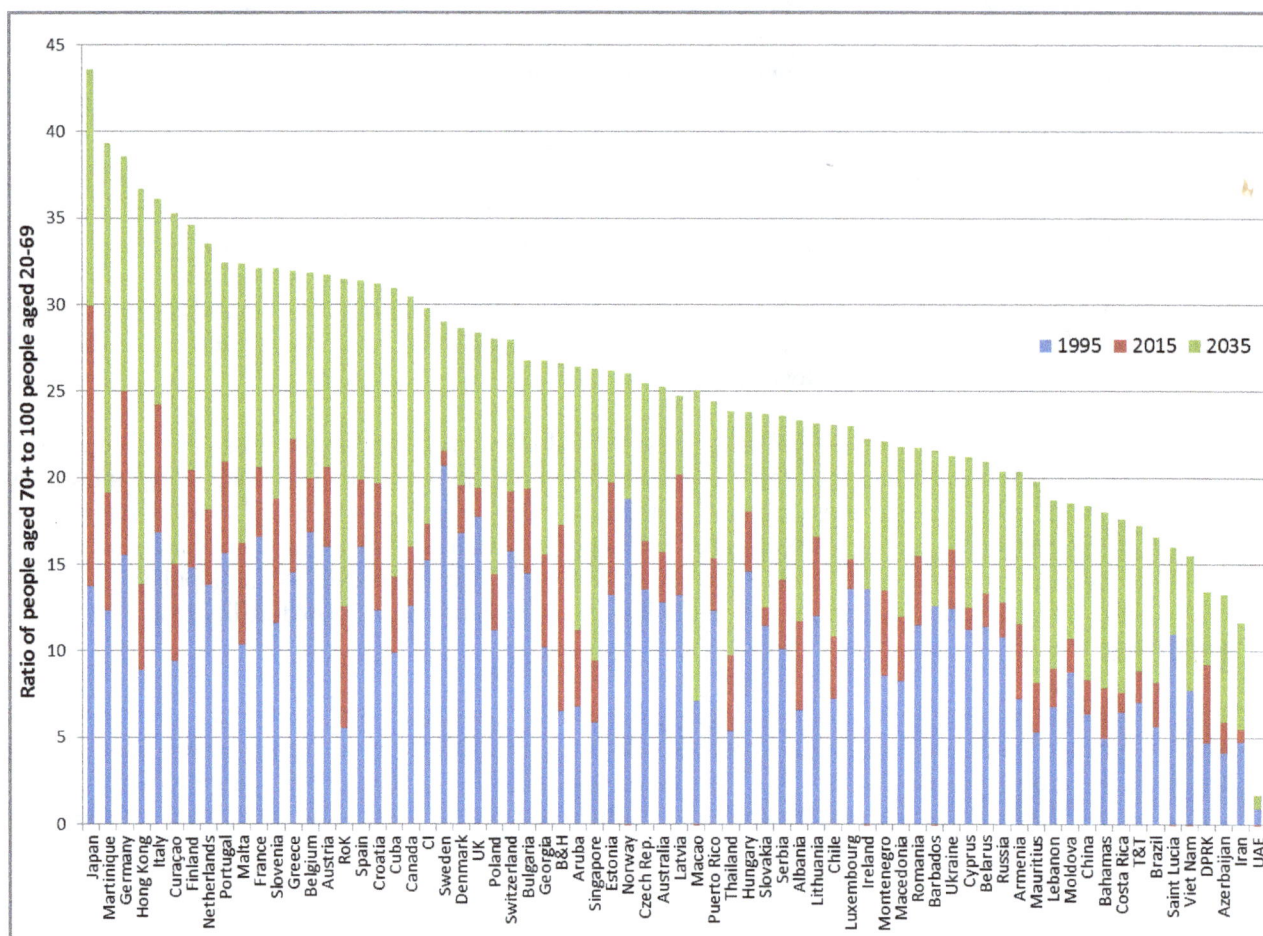

Source: United Nations, 2013a.
NOTES: CI refers to Channel Islands, DPRK refers to Democratic People's Republic of Korea, RoK refers to Republic of Korea; T&T refers to Trinidad and Tobago, UAE refers to United Arab Emirates, UK refers to United Kingdom.

G. POLICY APPROACHES TO LOW FERTILITY

Governments in many low-fertility countries have concerns over the implications of sustained low fertility, and governmental policies have shifted accordingly since around the time of the ICPD in 1994 (figure I.15). In 2013, a majority (about 70 per cent) of the 62 current low-fertility countries with data had a policy to raise fertility levels, an increase from just 30 per cent of those countries in 1996.[4] Of particular note are the low-fertility countries in Asia and Latin America and the Caribbean that had a policy to lower fertility in 1996 and that have since experienced very rapid fertility transitions. No low-fertility country had a policy to lower fertility in 2013. Given the different pathways to and characteristics of low fertility among countries, the consequences of low fertility levels and the nature of policy approaches adopted have varied as well.

---

[4] Serbia is included as Serbia and Montenegro in 1996. Montenegro also had a policy to raise fertility in 2013 but is excluded from the analysis.

While an increasing number of Governments are trying to raise fertility levels, early childbearing still characterizes a number of low-fertility countries. Policies to raise fertility or to prevent further fertility decline in these countries will need to focus on approaches relevant for older women due to the social and economic disadvantages associated with early childbearing and the relatively high rates of adolescent childbearing in some countries. Ireland and the United Kingdom stand out in Europe as they have a distinct "polarized" pattern of reproduction that includes high rates of childlessness and higher adolescent birth rates than comparable countries (Sobotka, 2013). High adolescent childbearing and socioeconomic inequalities among who bears children at young ages also continue to characterize many countries in Latin America and the Caribbean (Cavenaghi, 2013; Rodriguez-Vignoli and Cavenaghi, 2014). Policy interventions in these low-fertility countries still need to be strengthened in order to enable young people to prevent unintended pregnancy.

Figure I.15. Percentage of low-fertility countries with government policies on fertility levels by type of policy, 1996 and 2013

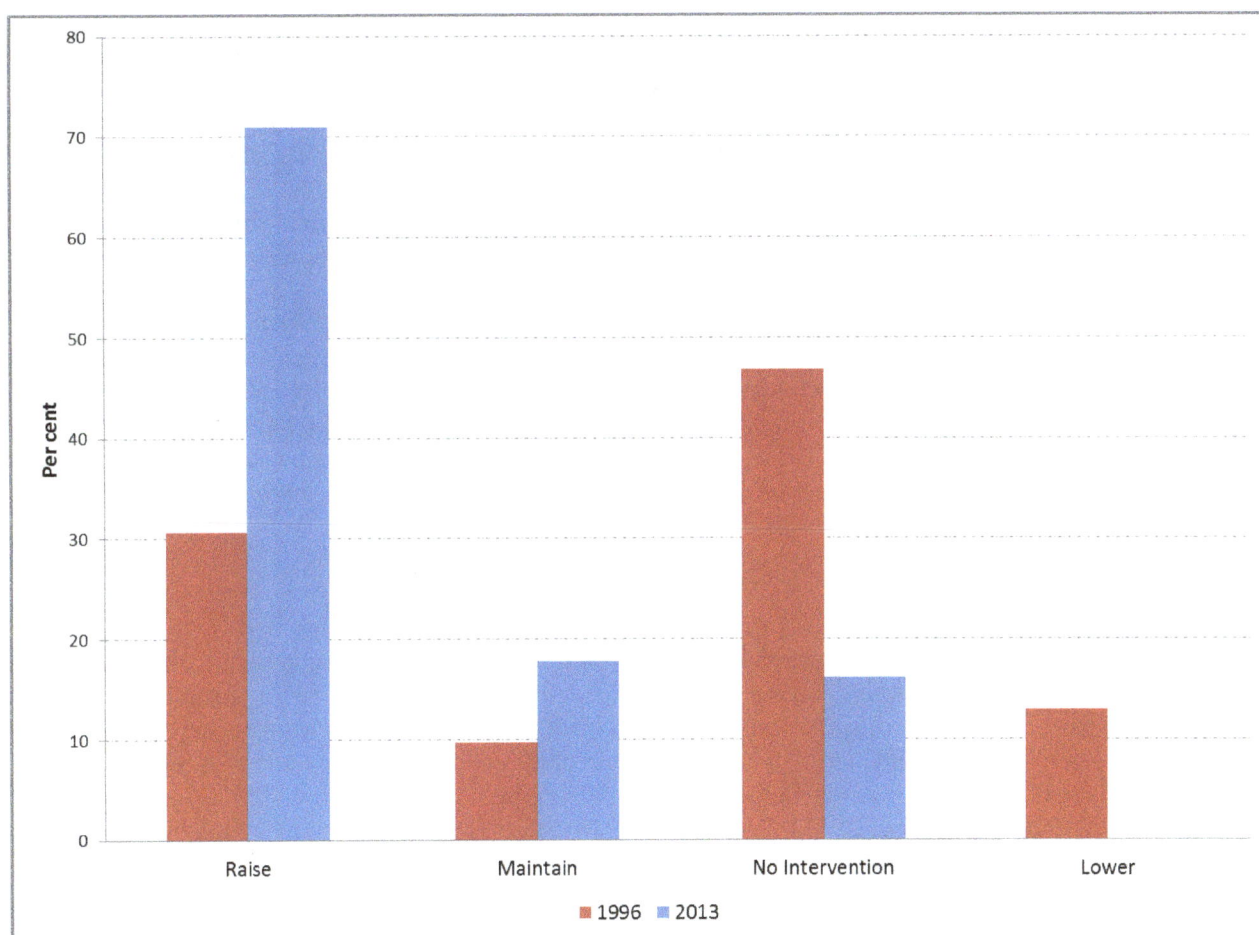

Source: United Nations (2013c).

1. *Pro-natalist policies*

The success of policies to influence fertility in low-fertility countries has not been impressive for the most part. Studies have shown a small but significant effect of national policies on fertility (Billingsley and Ferrarini, 2014). However, there is room for improvement in measuring the effects of policies and understanding the mechanisms involved (Gauthier, 2007; Gauthier, 2008), and long-term changes in fertility preferences could still emerge (Kohler and others, 2006; Stephen, 2012; Balbo and others, 2013). The wider context of social, cultural and economic factors in low-fertility countries seems to matter more for influencing fertility levels than specific policy interventions per se (Hoorens and others, 2011).

Interestingly, despite major shifts in family values and behaviours in Europe, the two-child family ideal has remained dominant, including among the most educated groups (Sobotka, 2013), and ideal family size is still close to replacement-level even in countries that experienced early declines in fertility to very low levels (Sobotka and Beaujouan, 2014). Furthermore, despite the very low fertility levels reached in Eastern and Southern Europe, childlessness has not been considered desirable, with most people expressing a desire for at least one child (Kohler and others, 2002). Thus, an effective policy will facilitate the conditions that best enable people to reach their desired family size (Sobotka, 2013).

Biological constraints to fecundity are an increasingly important factor as childbearing is postponed to older ages. Given that ideal family size has remained relatively stable, the postponement of childbearing means that desired family size may not be achieved, leading to a divergence of desired fertility and achieved fertility (Hoorens and others, 2011) or what has been termed "an unmet need for children" (Balbo and others, 2013). As a consequence, the demand for and use of assisted reproductive technology has grown. Reports of the European Society of Human Reproduction and Embryology covering 31 countries in Europe showed that medically assisted reproduction treatments (ART), including assisted reproductive technology cycles and intrauterine insemination cycles, have continued to increase year by year, reaching more than half a million of cycles in 2010 (Kupka and others, 2014). An analysis of 14 European countries with ART data over the period 1997 to 2009 showed that the proportion of births attributed to assisted reproduction has also grown over time, with the highest level observed in Demark (nearly 5 per cent of births in 2007) (Kocourkova and others, 2014).

2. *Financial incentives*

The evidence for the effect of financial incentives on increasing fertility is mixed and often temporary and transient (Hoorens and others, 2011). Financial incentives take different forms, including payments upon the birth of a baby, child allowances and tax breaks. In most countries, the payments are not sufficient to cover the direct and indirect costs of raising children and often have the most effect on either the lowest income families or larger families where the marginal cost of each child is lower (Thévenon and Gauthier, 2011; Thévenon, 2011). A study of 16 Western European countries found no significant effect of direct child allowances on either the timing of births or completed fertility (Kalwij, 2010). Generous child allowances in the United Kingdom were found to encourage young motherhood with little effect on overall fertility (Balbo and others, 2013). Where the financial incentives are particularly generous, such as in France or Quebec, Canada, there is evidence that there is a fertility benefit for higher income families as well (Thévenon, 2011). It appears that policies, which reduce the opportunity cost of having children seem to have a greater influence on fertility than direct financial incentives (Hoorens and others, 2011; Kalwij, 2010), although this influence varies by region and by country.

3. *Marriage*

Involuntary non-marriage has been implicated as a cause of childlessness mainly in low-fertility countries of Eastern Asia and South-Eastern Asia than in other regions (Jones, 2007), although a weakening of the desire to have children could, in turn, be responsible for decreased marriage rates (Jones, 2012). Low-fertility countries in Asia are generally characterised by low levels of adolescent childbearing, increasing levels of never-married women and childlessness, low levels of extra-marital childbearing and postponement of childbearing to later ages. The increase in never-married women in Asia particularly characterizes more-educated women (Jones, 2010). Policies to increase fertility need to consider whether postponement or rejection of marriage is a barrier to childbearing (Abbasi-Shavazi and Gubhaju, 2014; Jones, 2012; Stephen, 2012). Any policy to increase fertility in most low-fertility countries in Asia will also need to address barriers to marriage that may exist. Singapore is the only country that has explicitly focused on policies to increase marriage through housing policy and government matchmaking services with some limited success (Jones, 2012).

4. *Work-life balance*

The compatibility between childbearing and labour force participation, especially for women, is a key factor influencing fertility. Countries have taken different approaches to address this issue with varying success. Childcare subsidies seem to vary in impact depending on the broader social and economic context, the structure of childcare systems and the varying needs of parents (Gauthier and Philipov, 2008). For example, in countries with a culture of long working hours, the impact of subsidies for institutional childcare could be limited (Boling, 2008). In the Republic of Korea, where people work the longest hours of any Organization for Economic Cooperation and Development (OECD) country, there is also very limited public provision of childcare; nearly half of all employed women quit their jobs when they have children as parenthood and employment are particularly incompatible (Stephen, 2012). In the low-fertility countries in Eastern Asia, women face a stark choice between motherhood and a career due to a patriarchal environment and slow policy responses (Abbassi and Gubhaju, 2014; Frejka and others, 2010).

Japan and Singapore have focused on policies promoting marriage and childbearing through direct subsidies for childbearing and more family-friendly policies like subsidized childcare and paid maternity leave. The Republic of Korea also supported subsidized childcare and parental leave but not direct support for childbearing (Abbassi and Gubhaju, 2014). However, in none of these countries have the policies had much success in influencing fertility as fertility has continued to decline to very low levels with low-fertility Eastern Asian countries often presenting women with a stark choice between motherhood and a career due to a patriarchal environment and slow policy responses (Abbassi and Gubhaju 2014; Frejka and others 2010). In contrast, in other OECD countries, the provision of childcare services for children under the age of three was found to be a more effective policy lever for increasing fertility than other factors such as leave entitlements and benefits granted around childbirth (Luci-Greulich and Thévenon, 2013). For the provision of childcare to work effectively to influence fertility, the provision of childcare services must be available at the appropriate times and continuously over the childhood period. In that respect, countries in Eastern Europe and Southern Europe as well as Japan and the Republic of Korea lag behind other OECD countries (Thévenon, 2011). Childcare policies in Singapore appear to partially account for why fertility is higher there as compared with other similar Eastern Asian countries (Jones, 2012).

Strong support for work-life balance seems to support higher fertility (Kalwij, 2010) with different policy models leading to higher fertility in Nordic and Anglo-Saxon countries (Andersson, 2008; Thévenon, 2011). In Nordic countries, the work-life balance is achieved through significant State interventions. Anglo-Saxon countries tend to see part-time work of parents (mainly mothers) with young children as a private choice but taxes are still structured in order to provide support for this option (Thévenon, 2011). In contrast, in Southern European countries, the strong family orientation seems to drive fertility downwards with little public policy attention to being able to combine parenthood with work or education (Hoorens and others, 2011).

There is mixed evidence on the effect of parental leave on fertility and this varies greatly across countries depending on the nature of the leave (Hoorens and others, 2011; Thévenon, 2011). In Nordic countries, there is evidence that where fathers take parental leave, there are more second- and third-order births (Duvander and others, 2010). Research in Sweden has shown that parental-leave allowance reduces the postponement of births (Balbo and others, 2013).

On the whole, Nordic and Western European countries have been the most successful in adapting to low fertility with family-friendly policies, increased childcare availability, and increased and more flexible parental leave, including for fathers (Balbo and others, 2013; Kalwij, 2010; Thévenon, 2011). Although direct attribution is difficult to establish, these countries have also been most successful in avoiding lowest-low fertility levels.

In sum, policies designed to increase fertility have had only limited success. Given the varying pathways to low fertility and the social, economic and institutional environment in which fertility behaviour occurs, countries should tailor policies to their specific contexts (Luci-Greulich and Thevenon, 2013). One unifying factor that emerges is the importance of gender equity in influencing fertility. Gender inequity affects the ability of mothers to combine working and parenthood, when women disproportionately carry the burden of childcare and household maintenance. Public policies can mitigate some of these effects, such as through the provision of paternal leave and accessible and affordable childcare, although other effects, especially at the household and individual level, are less amenable to direct government intervention.

II. HIGH FERTILITY

Since the International Conference on Population and Development (ICPD) in 1994, fertility has continued to fall in many countries and regions in the world. However, fertility still remains considerably above replacement level in a significant number of countries, predominantly in sub-Saharan Africa. Trends in high-fertility countries are important to understand as these countries are increasingly responsible for the largest portion of global population growth. Furthermore, most high-fertility countries are also low-income countries, where a growing and youthful population challenges the public provision of basic services such as for education and health.

In this report, high fertility is defined as a period total fertility level greater than 3.2 children per woman in 2005-2010. Among the 66 high-fertility countries, fertility is highest in Eastern Africa, Middle Africa and Western Africa where total fertility is above five children per woman in the majority of high-fertility countries (figure II.1). Fertility, while still high, is much lower in countries of Asia, Latin America and the Caribbean, Southern Africa and Oceania, where many countries included in this report as high-fertility countries, have a total fertility below four children per woman.

A. CHANGES IN TOTAL FERTILITY AND AGE-SPECIFIC FERTILITY RATES

1. *Maximum fertility and onset of fertility decline*

High-fertility countries vary in the timing and speed of fertility decline. The transition from maximum fertility experienced since 1950 to the lowest fertility level (figure II.2) was very steep in many countries, with the steepest transitions predominantly in regions outside of Europe.[5] In the majority of high-fertility countries, the maximum fertility reached (the red square markers on the line graphs in figure II.2) was seven or more children per woman. Only among countries in Middle Africa, Northern Africa, Southern Africa and Latin America and the Caribbean was maximum fertility below seven children per woman. There were wide variations in maximum fertility in Eastern Africa, Middle Africa and Asia compared to other regions. Most high-fertility countries in Africa reached maximum fertility much later, after 1975, compared to countries in other regions. All the high-fertility countries in Latin America and the Caribbean experienced maximum fertility by the mid-1960s, as did most high-fertility countries in Oceania (figure II.2).

Fertility decline had already begun in most high-fertility countries by the time of the 1994 ICPD (the date of the onset of fertility decline is shown by the green round marker for each country in figure II.2; the vertical line marks 1994). All high-fertility countries in Latin America and the Caribbean and Oceania and 80 per cent of high-fertility countries in Asia had begun the fertility transition by 1994, whereas only one in three countries in Middle Africa and about half of countries in Eastern and Western Africa had done so. Among the 23 high-fertility countries not in transition at the time of the 1994 ICPD, most have since entered a fertility transition; by 2010, only three countries have not yet done so and all are in Western Africa (Gambia, Mali and Niger).

---

[5] Maximum fertility is defined in this report as the highest level of period total fertility reached since 1950. The onset of fertility decline is defined as the first year in which there is 10 per cent decline in fertility from maximum fertility and where fertility levels do not return to maximum fertility levels (Coale, 1986).

Figure II.1 Levels of total fertility in high-fertility countries, 2005-2010

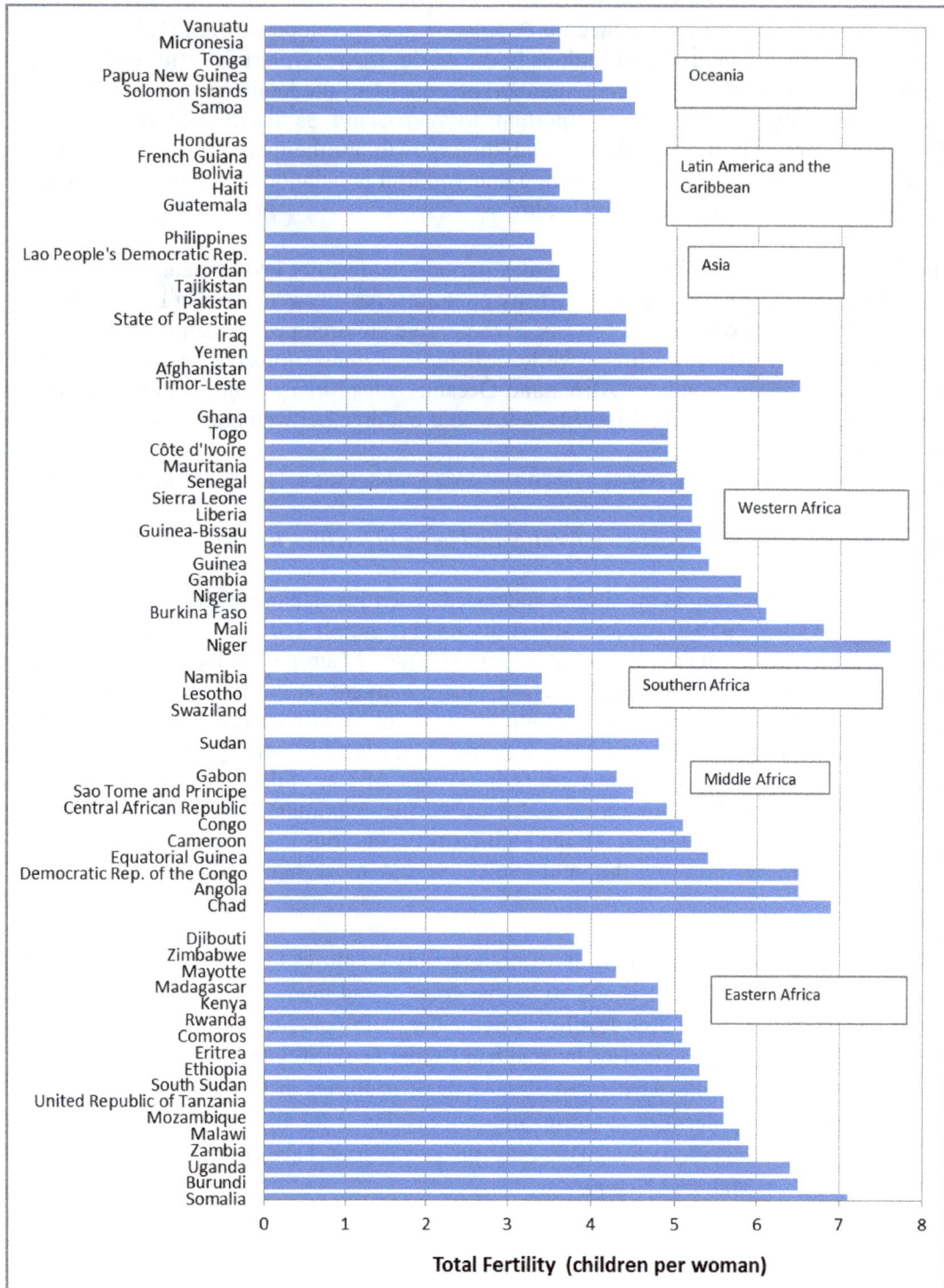

Total Fertility (children per woman)

Source: United Nations (2013a).

Figure II.2. Maximum fertility and onset of fertility decline among high-fertility countries

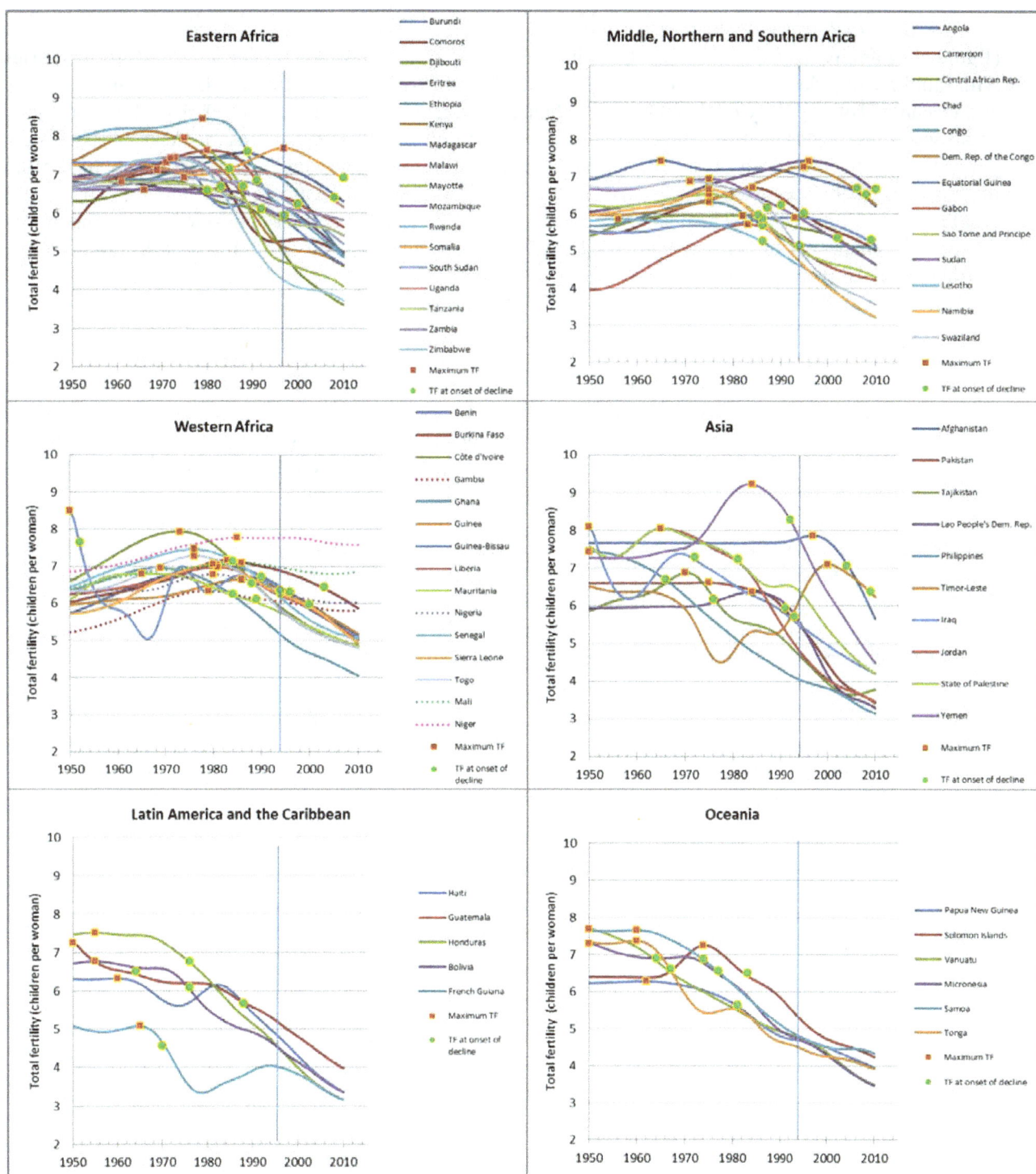

Source: United Nations (2013a).
NOTE: The date at which maximum fertility was reached in each country is shown in annex table 5 and by the red square markers on the line graphs in figure II.2.

2. Pace of fertility decline since the 1994 ICPD

The pace of fertility decline varied greatly across the high-fertility countries since the 1994 ICPD (figure II.3, annex table 6). Some declines have been rapid and substantial. The high-fertility countries with rapid fertility declines are predominantly in Asia, Latin America and the Caribbean, Southern Africa and Oceania. Total fertility declined by more than 25 per cent between 1994 and 2010 in almost as many countries in Africa (Djibouti, Ethiopia, Lesotho, Namibia and Swaziland) as in Asia (Afghanistan, Pakistan, Lao People's Democratic Republic, Jordan, State of Palestine and Yemen). Substantial fertility declines since 1994 occurred in Yemen (43 per cent), Lao People's Democratic Republic (41 per cent) and Pakistan (38 per cent). The decline in Yemen is even more extraordinary considering that maximum fertility in Yemen was an extremely high 9.2 children per woman in 1980-1985. In Latin America and the Caribbean, fertility declined by more than 25 per cent since 1994 in Bolivia, Guatemala, Haiti and Honduras. Total fertility declined to under four children per woman in the majority of countries that experienced rapid decline.

Moderate declines in fertility, between 15 and 25 per cent, occurred in most countries in Western Africa and a few countries in Eastern Africa, Central Africa, Asia and Oceania (middle panel in figure II.3). Total fertility declined by more than 20 per cent in Eritrea, Madagascar, Rwanda and South Sudan (in Eastern Africa); Benin, Ghana, Guinea-Bissau and Sierra Leone (in Western Africa); Iraq, Philippines and Tajikistan (in Asia); and French Guiana, Solomon Islands and Sudan.

Fertility decline in other high-fertility countries has been stalled since the 1994 ICPD, where fertility has begun to decline but the pace of decline has decreased or stopped altogether (Bongaarts and Casterline, 2012; Ezeh and others, 2012). Total fertility declined by less than 15 per cent between 1994 and 2010 in most high-fertility countries in Eastern Africa and Middle Africa. Fertility decline was slowest or appears to have stalled in Congo, Gambia, Kenya, Mali, Niger, Nigeria, Samoa, Tanzania, Timor-Leste and Zambia. Among these countries, the onset of fertility decline has not begun in Gambia, Mali and Niger; in others, the fertility transition started before 1994 in Congo (1986), Kenya (1982), Samoa (1974), Tanzania (1992) and Zambia (1987). Timor-Leste is the country where the fertility transition began most recently (2009).

Figure II.3. Fertility decline in high-fertility countries from 1994 to 2010

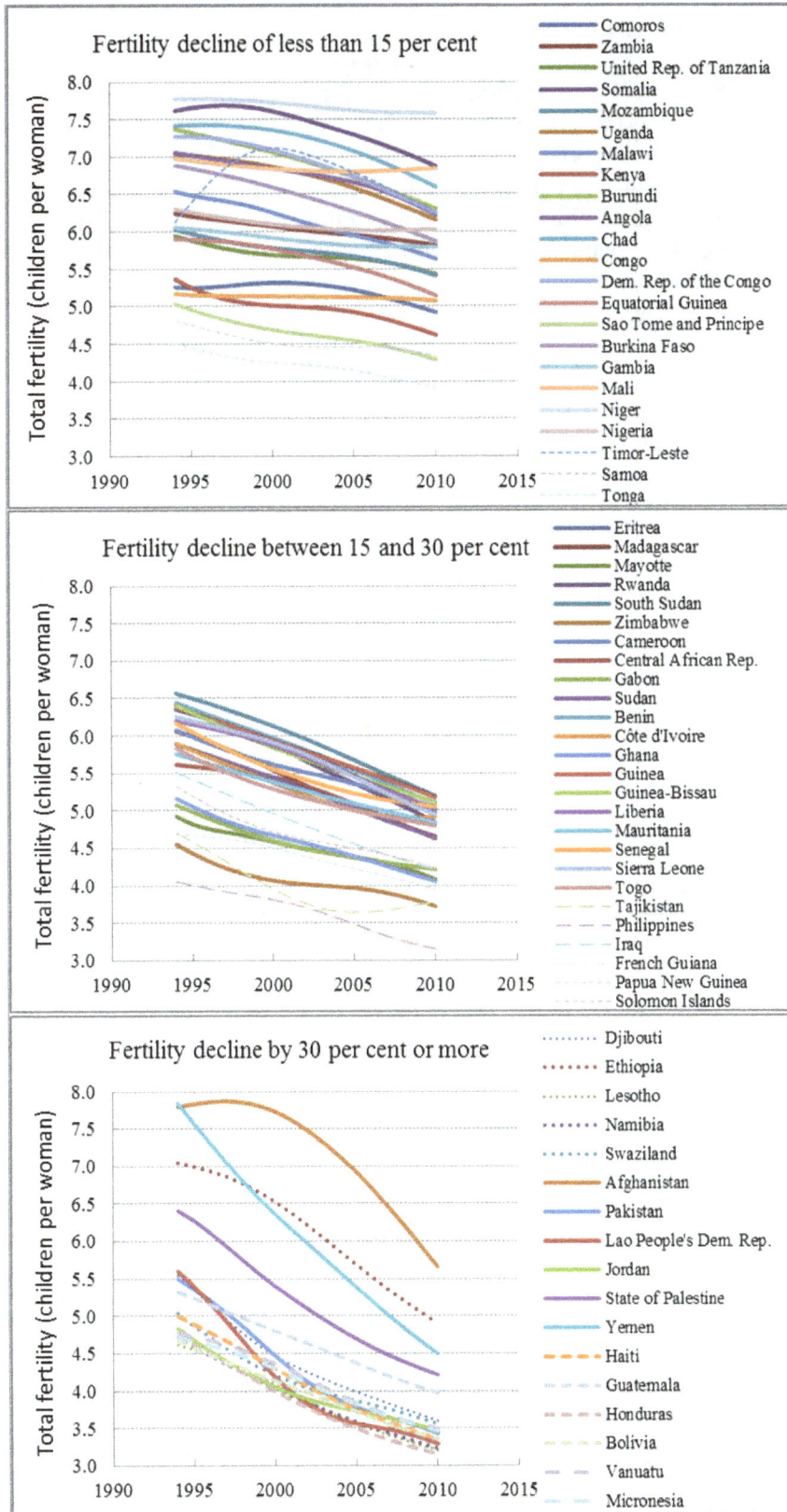

Source: United Nations (2013a).

3. *Fertility decline at young and old ages*

Fertility decline is not usually uniform across all age groups, and changes in fertility at the youngest and oldest reproductive age groups are especially important for demographic, social and health reasons. The adolescent birth rate (ABR) is of particular interest given the serious impact that early pregnancy has on the lives of young women (United Nations, 2013d). Moreover, reducing adolescent pregnancy and childbearing continues to be an important objective for Governments (United Nations, 2013c). Women, at the other extreme of the reproductive period, aged 40 years and older, are also of note as there are public health concerns regarding births to older women. For example, maternal mortality rates tend to be higher when mothers are 40 years or over (Blanc and others, 2013; World Bank, 2010). Moreover, fertility declines are often led by fertility limitation behaviour among women at older ages who have completed their families (Sneeringer, 2009).

Most high-fertility countries experienced a decline in the adolescent birth rate (the average number of births per 1,000 women aged 15-19 years) between 1990-1995 and 2005-2010 (countries below the red line in figure II.4). In four countries, the adolescent birth rate declined by 50 per cent or more (countries below the dashed red line). In contrast, adolescent fertility increased since 1990-1995 in eight countries; this increase was relatively small (11 per cent or less) in Iraq, Lesotho, Philippines and Timor-Leste but relatively large (20 per cent or more) in Mayotte, Mozambique, Somalia and Zambia.

Figure II.4. Adolescent birth rates in 1990-1995 and 2005-2010, high-fertility countries

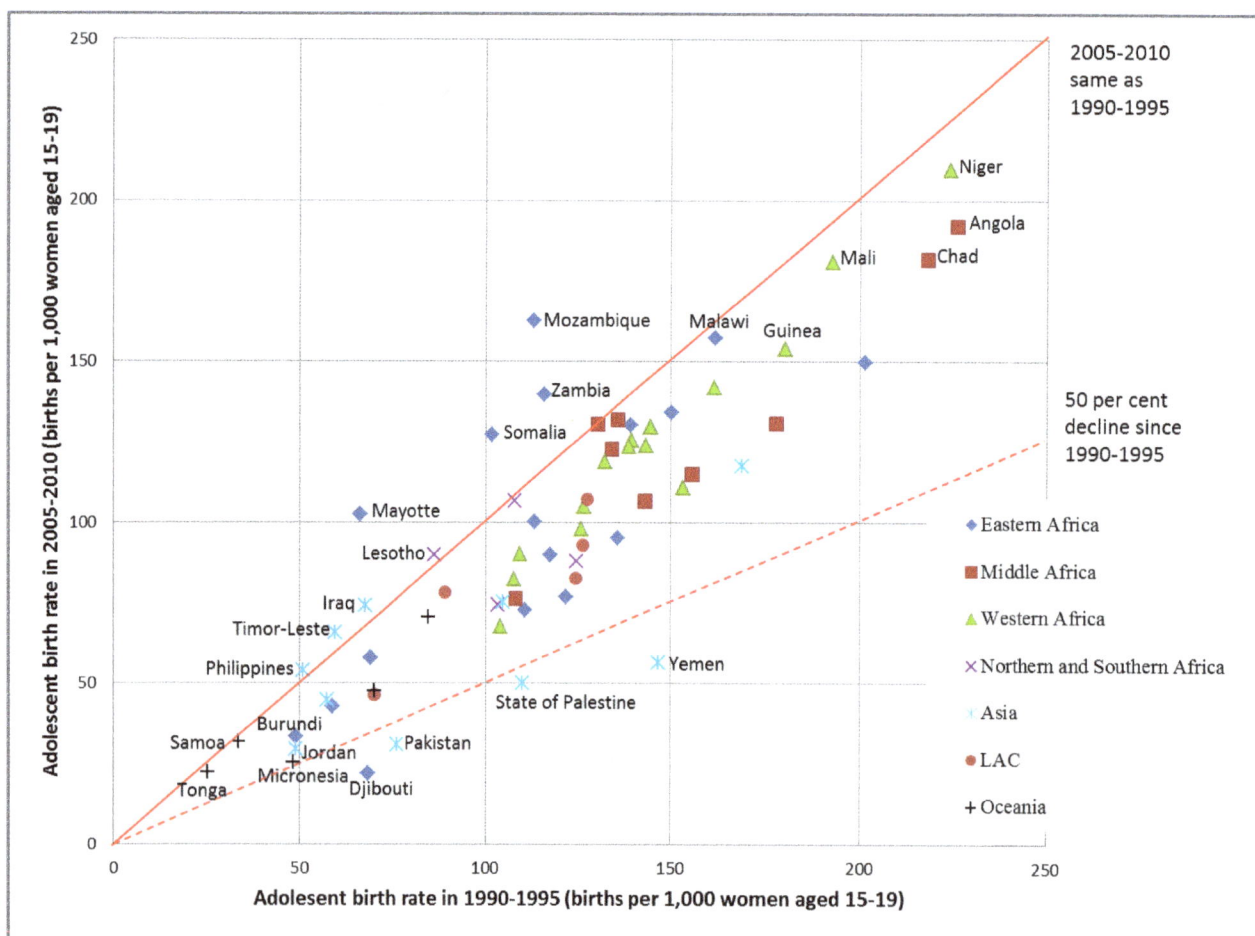

Source: United Nations (2013a).
NOTE: LAC refers to Latin America and the Caribbean

Countries with persistently high adolescent birth rates are concentrated mainly in Middle Africa and Western Africa. Angola, Chad, Mali and Niger had the highest adolescent birth rates in 2005-2010 (more than 180 births per 1,000 women aged 15-19) despite declines since 1990-1995. Even within the same region, adolescent birth rates vary widely among high-fertility countries. In Eastern Africa, for example, Burundi, Djibouti and Rwanda have adolescent birth rates below 50 births per 1,000 women aged 15-19 while Malawi, Mozambique and Uganda have high rates of 150 births or more per 1,000 women aged 15-19 years.

The fertility of older women, measured as the age-specific fertility rate of women aged 40-44 years has dramatically declined, in many high-fertility countries since the 1994 ICPD (figure II.5). In Lao People's Democratic Republic, Namibia and Pakistan, fertility among older women declined by 50 per cent or more since 1990-1995 (countries below the red dashed line in figure II.5). By 2005-2010, only four high-fertility countries (Gambia, Papua New Guinea, Tajikistan and Timor-Leste) had birth rates among older women higher than levels in 1990-1995. Nonetheless, fertility among older women remains high in many countries in Eastern Africa and Western Africa, including Burundi, Mali, Niger, Rwanda and Somalia where more than 100 births per 1,000 women aged 40-44 years occurred in 2005-2010.

Figure II.5. Birth rate of women aged 40-44 years in 1990-1995 and 2005-2010, high-fertility countries

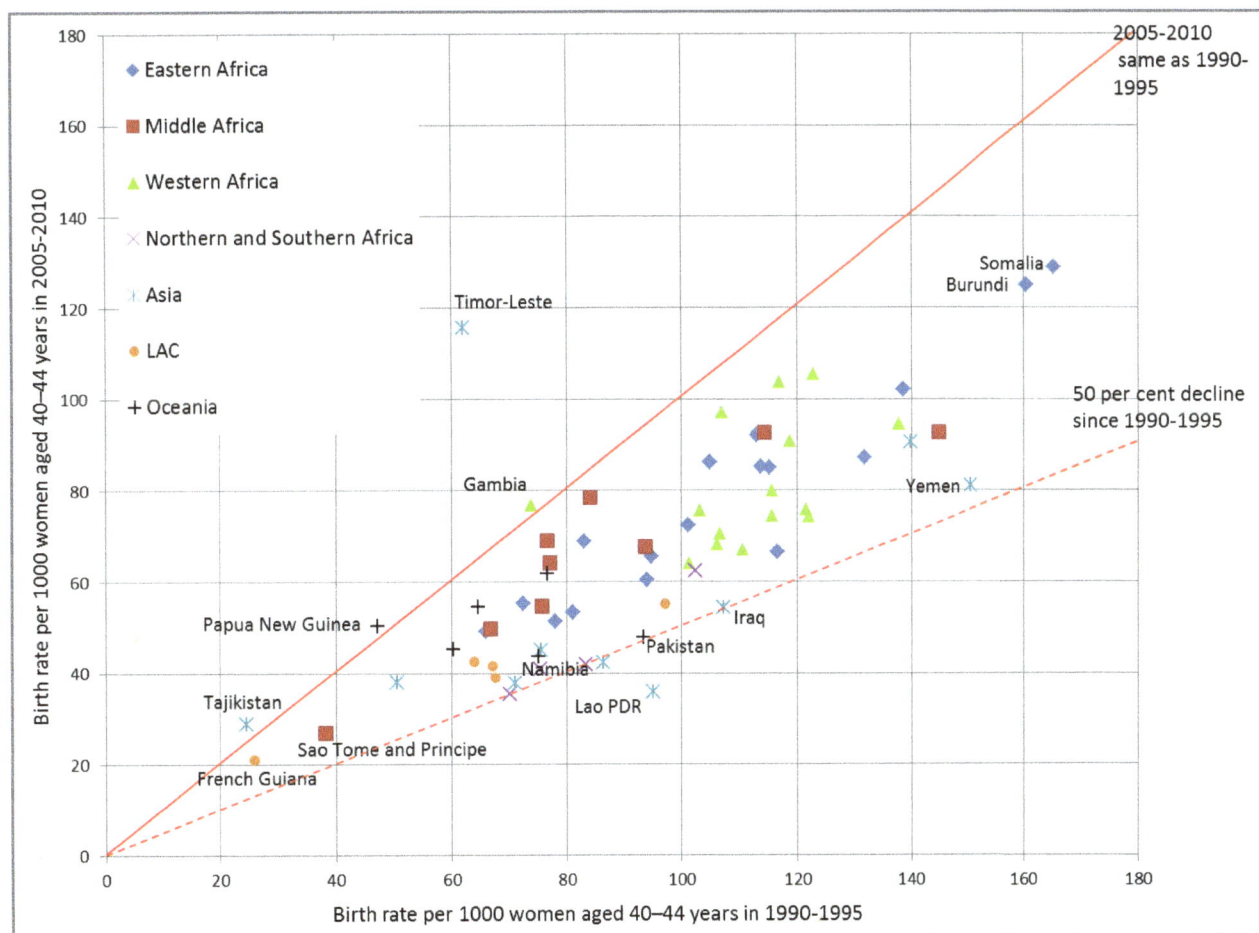

Source: United Nations (2013a).

The decline in fertility among older women surpassed the decline in the adolescent birth rate in many countries. Between 1990-1995 and 2005-2010, the decline in fertility among women aged 40-44 years (the red bars in figure II.6) was equal to or more than the decline in the adolescent birth rate in 11 of the 45 high-fertility countries in Africa (Burundi, Central African Republic, Djibouti, Eritrea, Gabon, Gambia, Nigeria, Rwanda, Sao Tome and Principe, South Sudan and Zimbabwe); half of the high-fertility countries in Asia (Pakistan, State of Palestine, Tajikistan and Yemen), and in all countries in Oceania except Samoa and Tonga. Timor-Leste is in a distinctive position because the fertility of both younger and older women increased over this time period.

Figure II.6. Percentage change in the birth rates of adolescents and women aged 40-44 years between 1990-1995 and 2005-2010, high-fertility countries

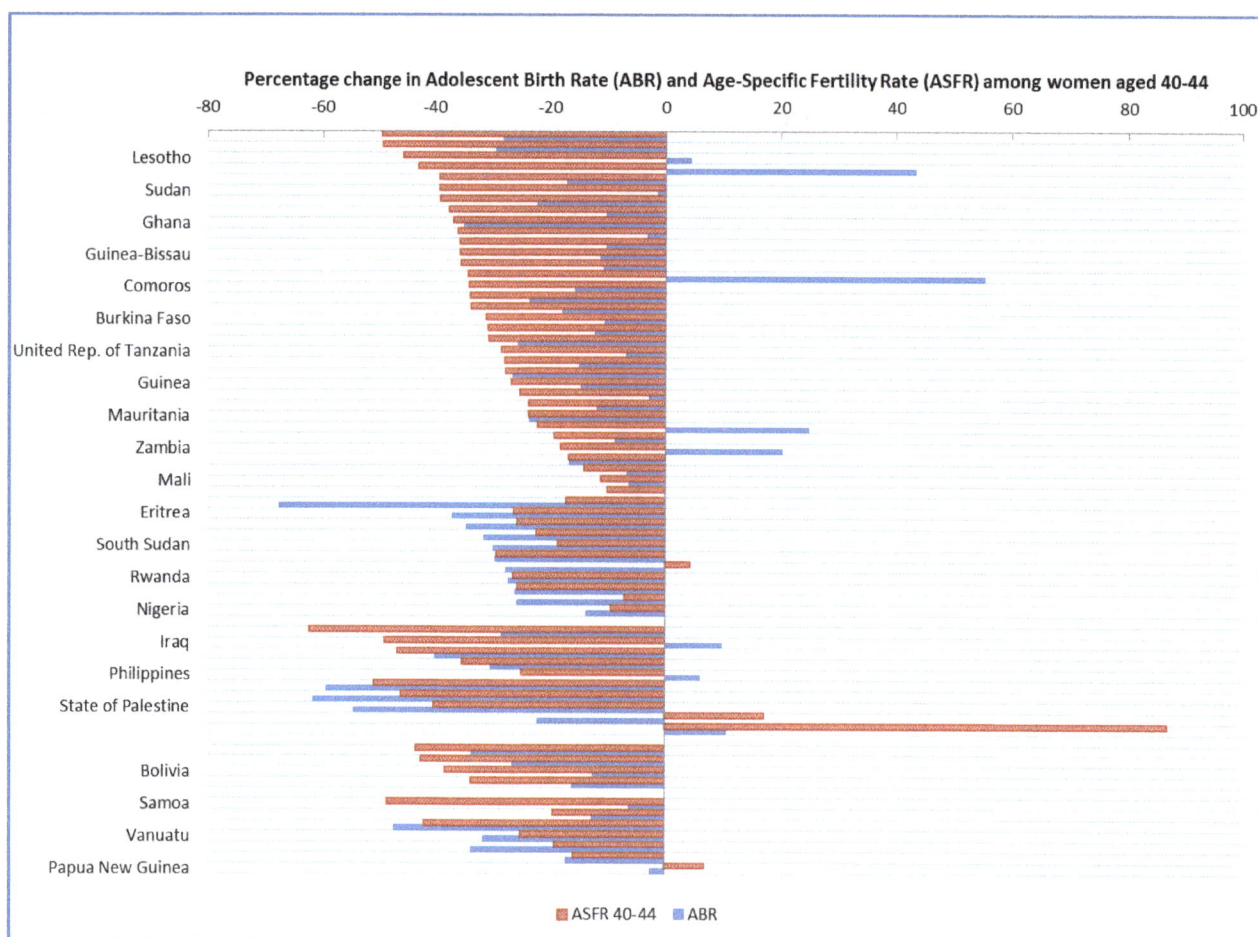

Percentage change in Adolescent Birth Rate (ABR) and Age-Specific Fertility Rate (ASFR) among women aged 40-44

■ ASFR 40-44   ■ ABR

Source: United Nations (2013a).

How much of the decline (or increase) in total fertility is accounted for by fertility changes among younger and older women? The proportion of total fertility decline that is attributable to the decline in adolescent fertility is calculated by dividing the change in the adolescent fertility rate between 1990-1995 and 2005-2010 by the change in total fertility over the same period. Similarly, the proportion of total fertility decline that is attributable to the decline in the fertility of older women is calculated by dividing the change in the age-specific fertility rate of women aged 40-44 years between 1990-1995 and 2005-2010 by the change in period total fertility over the same period.

In the majority of high-fertility countries, fertility decline among older women accounts for a larger proportion of the decline in total fertility than the decline in ABR (figure II.7). Countries where a large proportion of total fertility decline is attributed to the decline in ABR are also countries where the decline in total fertility was small between 1990-1995 and 2005-2010. This is the case in countries such as Angola, Chad, Mali, Niger, Nigeria and Uganda, where a relatively small decline in the adolescent birth rate accounted for between 25 and 40 per cent of the overall decline in total fertility. In Gambia, the decline in adolescent fertility accounted for a 72 per cent decline in total fertility despite the relative stall in fertility change between 1994 and 2010 (figure II.3). In a number of countries, the contribution of adolescent fertility was negative. In other words, total fertility declined due to declining fertility at older ages and despite an increase in the adolescent birth rate.

In high-fertility countries where the decline in total fertility has been small, a large proportion of the fertility decline is attributed to declines in fertility among both younger and older women. Fertility change among younger women aged 15-19 years and older women aged 40-44 years accounts for 88 per cent of the decline in total fertility in Comoros, 67 per cent in Gambia and 86 per cent in Niger between 1990-1995 and 2005-2010. In Angola, Chad, Mali, Nigeria, Uganda and Tanzania, 40-60 per cent of the decline in total fertility is attributed to fertility declines in these two age groups.

In most high-fertility countries, the decline in fertility among older women contributed to at least 10 per cent of the overall decline in total fertility since 1990-1995 (figure II.7). Among 33 high-fertility countries, fertility decline among older women contributed to 20 per cent or more of the fertility decline during this period and in 5 of these countries, over 50 per cent of the decline. Where the decline in the fertility of older women contributed disproportionately to the overall decline in total fertility, the age-specific fertility rates of younger women often increased over this period. Fertility in these countries could have declined further had there been concurrent declines in adolescent fertility.

Figure II.7. Percentage decline in total fertility attributed to change in birth rates among women aged 15-19 years and 40-44 years, 1990-1995 to 2005-2010, high-fertility countries

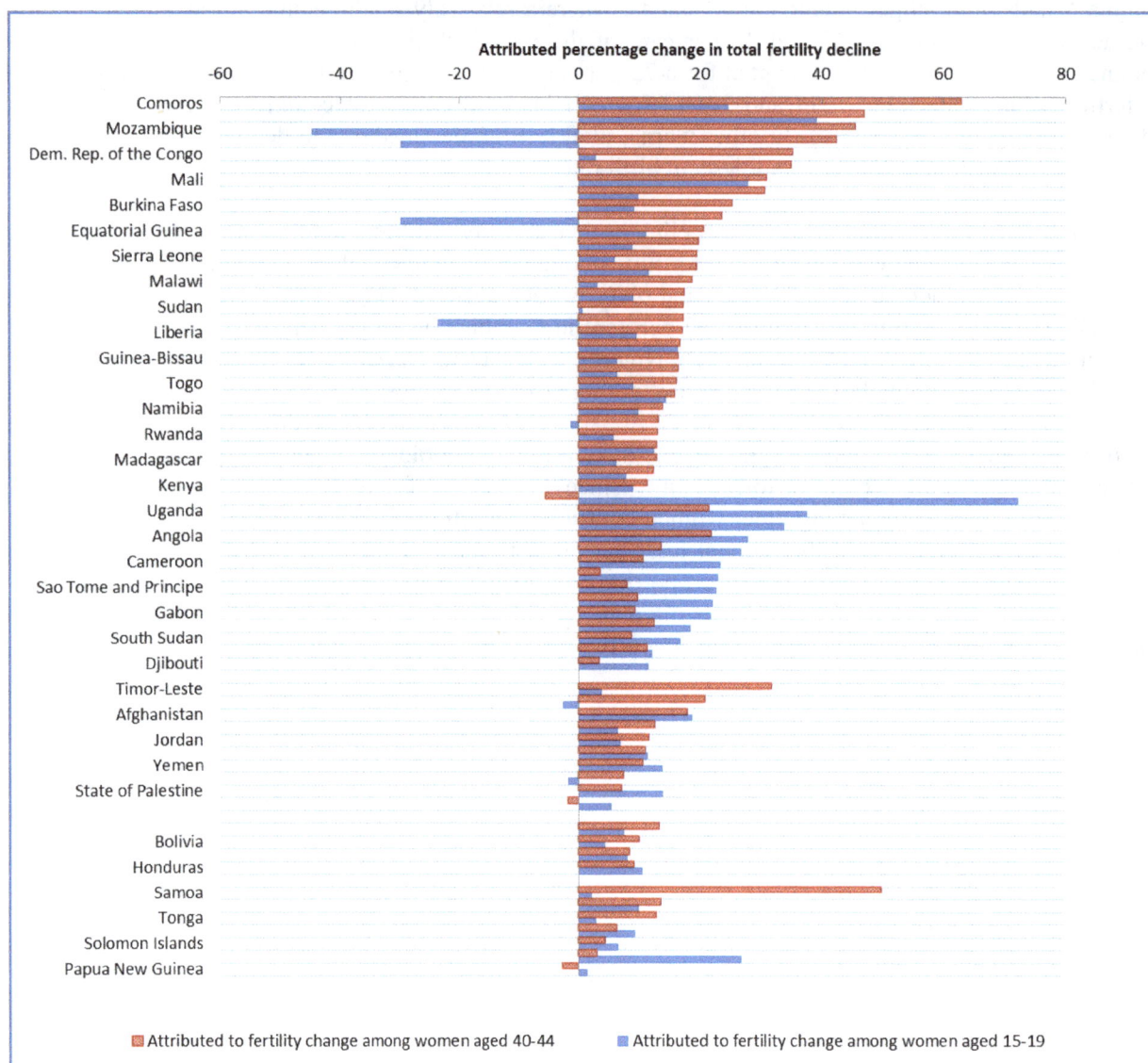

Source: United Nations (2013a).

B. FERTILITY PROJECTIONS

Projections of total fertility until 2030-2035 reflect the anticipated time period for the post-2015 development agenda and the approximate length of a generation in high-fertility countries from 2005-2010. Fertility changes in this period have implications for future population size as well (Andreev and others, 2013; United Nations, 2013a). Fertility projections are based on historical fertility trends of a given country and of all countries that have already experienced a fertility decline (United Nations, 2014b). Under the medium fertility variant, all high-fertility countries are projected to experience a decrease in fertility (figure II.8). In some countries, particularly those in Asia, the projected fertility decline is sharp. For example, total fertility in Afghanistan is projected to decline from 6.3 in 2005-2010 to 2.5 by 2030-2035, a decrease of more than 50 per cent. Timor-Leste and Yemen also have steep projected declines in total fertility.

Yet some of the highest fertility countries, particularly in Western African (Gambia, Mali, Niger and Nigeria), are projected to experience a decline of less than 25 per cent in total fertility by 2030-2035. The only countries with projected total fertility above four children per woman by 2030-2035 are in Eastern Africa, Middle Africa and Western Africa. Niger and Mali are projected to be global outliers with significantly higher fertility rates (more than 5.5 children per woman) than any other country. No high-fertility country is projected to reach below-replacement level fertility by 2030-2035.

Figure II.8. Total fertility for countries, 2005-2010 and projections for 2030-2035, high-fertility countries

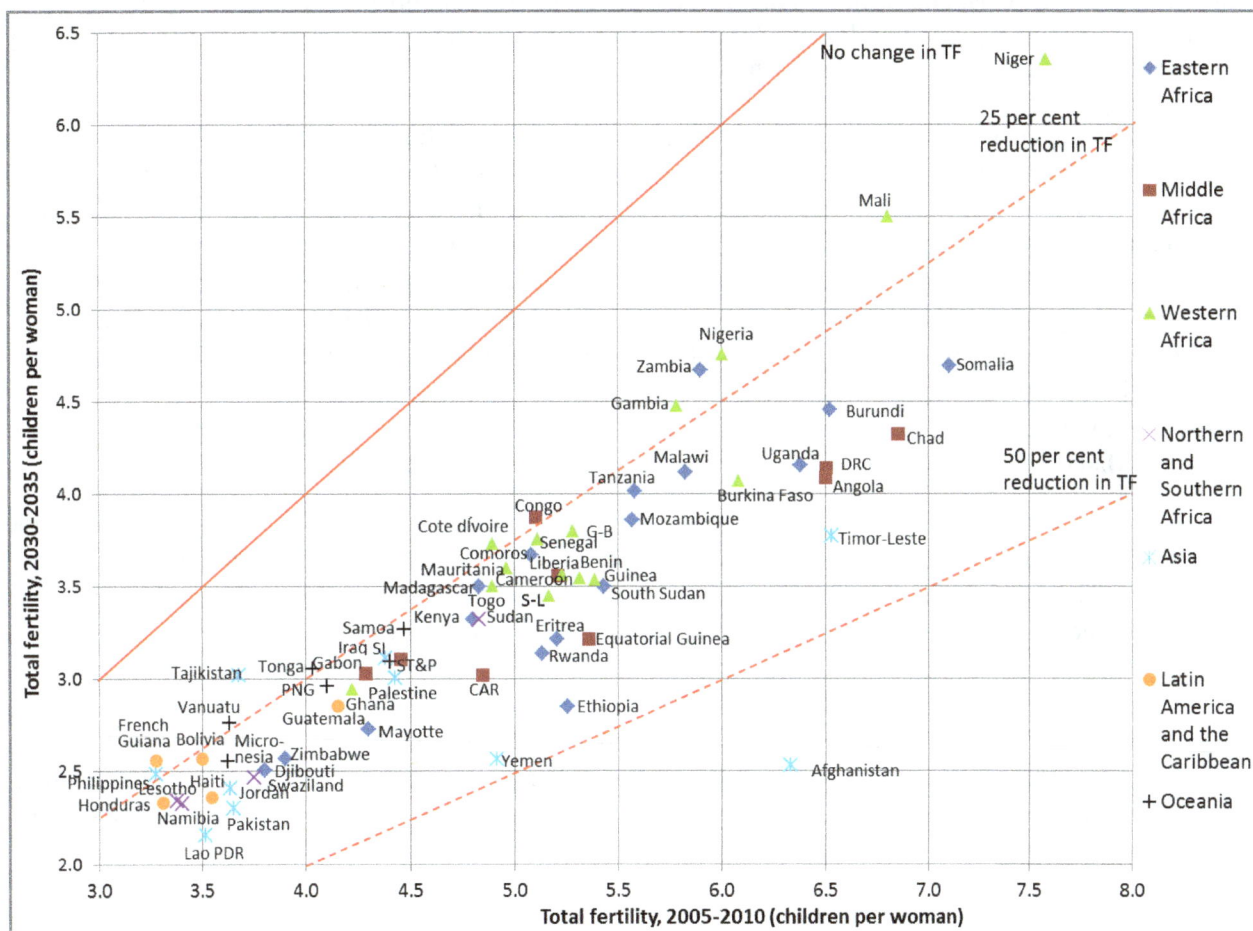

Source: United Nations (2013a) from medium fertility variant.
NOTES: CAR refers to Central African Republic, GB refers to Guinea-Bissau, SL refers to Sierra Leone, PNG refers to Papua New Guinea, ST&P refers to Sao Tome and Principe, SI refers to Solomon Islands.

C. CHANGES IN FERTILITY TIMING, MARRIAGE AND CONTRACEPTIVE USE

Many factors have contributed to the decline in fertility in high-fertility countries. These factors can be divided into broad cultural, economic and social factors, such as education or economic growth, that affect fertility through changes in proximate determinants such as marriage and sexual unions, breastfeeding, sterility, abortion and contraceptive use. A thorough consideration of all these factors is beyond the scope of this report. Instead, the focus is on changes in key correlates of fertility decline for which adequate data are currently available: age at first marriage, age at first birth, contraceptive use and unmet need for family planning (limiting and spacing).

1. *Age at first marriage and first birth*

In the majority of high-fertility countries, women are increasingly postponing first marriage to older ages. Age at first marriage represents for many women, the first exposure to the risk of pregnancy and childbearing. As a result, a younger age of marriage is associated with higher fertility rates as well as broader social, economic and health problems resulting from child and early marriage. Mean age at first birth marks the entry into motherhood and has risen in most countries, although the mean age at first birth still remains relatively young in countries in sub-Saharan Africa, especially Western Africa. In addition to the demographic, social and health issues surrounding adolescent childbearing (United Nations 2013d), a younger woman is exposed to a longer childbearing period if her first birth occurs early and she is likely to bear more children than if her first birth occurs later.

The female mean age at first marriage is generally increasing in high-fertility countries (first panel of figure II.9 and annex table 7).[6] Of the 29 high-fertility countries with available data, 27 had an increase in the female mean age at first marriage although overall regional trends are unclear. Still, the mean age at first marriage was less than 20 years in 18 countries according to the most recent data available (around 2009), down from 21 countries in the 1990s. Many countries in Middle Africa and Western Africa still had particularly young ages at first marriage fort the latest data point available. Six countries had a mean age at first marriage of less than 18 years for the latest point available, compared with 11 countries in the 1990s. The countries with the largest absolute increase in the mean age at first marriage are Eritrea, Gabon and Ghana, where the mean age at first marriage increased by 1.4 years per decade. In only one country, Madagascar, the female mean age at first marriage decreased over this time period.

There has also been an increase in the mean age at first birth in many high-fertility countries since the time of the ICPD (second panel of figure II.9 and annex table 7). Although countries in Middle Africa and Western Africa tend to have lower mean ages at first birth, many countries in this region have had substantial increases over time in the mean age at first birth. The increases in Eastern Africa and Southern Africa and in Latin America and the Caribbean have been more modest with Eritrea and Madagascar even experiencing a decrease in the mean age at first birth. Rwanda stands out as having a particularly high mean age at first birth for the region (22.9 years in 2010). The four high-fertility countries in Asia with data continue to have much older mean ages at first birth (22 years or older). Nonetheless, of the 29 high-fertility countries with data, the mean age at first birth was below 20 years for 19 countries in the 1990s and in 14 countries for the most recent year (since 2001).

The relationship between fertility change and the female mean age at first marriage and mean age at first birth shows that the adolescent birth rate has decreased as the mean age at first marriage and the mean age at first birth have increased in most countries with available data (figure II.9). Two exceptions are Mozambique and Zambia (the red arrows pointing upward), where the adolescent birth rate increased despite increases in the mean age at first marriage and mean age at first birth. While there is a general association between older ages at first marriage and first birth and lower levels of adolescent childbearing, the association is weak between older ages at marriage and trends in total fertility (Garenne, 2014).

---

[6] For 28 out of the 29 countries included in this analysis, the mean age at first marriage is based on national household surveys (mainly Demographic and Health Surveys) using the median age at first marriage for women aged 25-29 years. Because the data are drawn from surveys, a range of dates is used with the closest point to 1994 (from 1990-2000) and the latest point available (from 2001-2013).

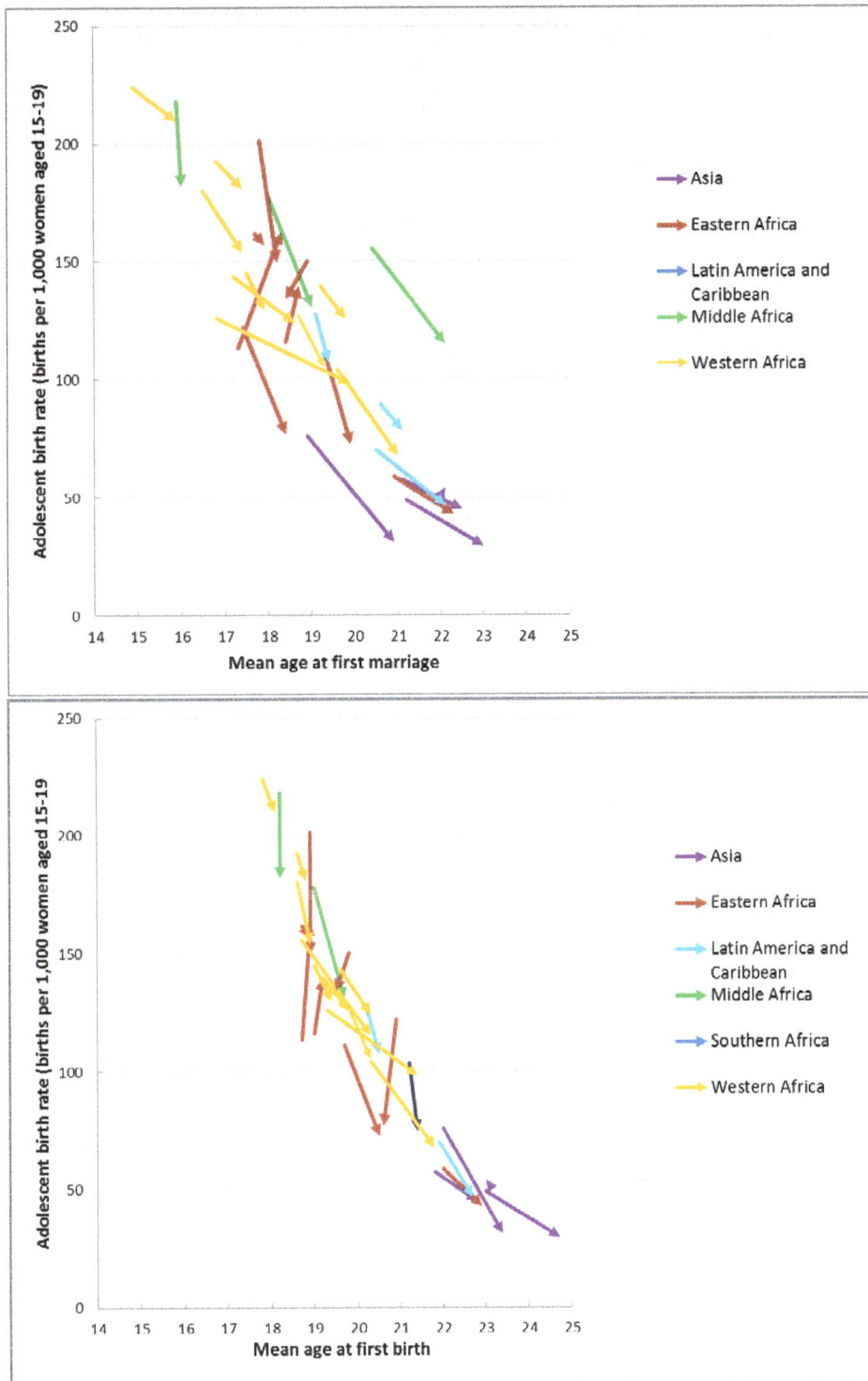

Figure II.9. Adolescent birth rate and mean age at first marriage and first birth, selected high-fertility countries, 1990s to latest data available

Source: Demographic and Health Surveys 1990-2013; see annex table 7.

2. Contraceptive prevalence

One of the main determinants of fertility is contraceptive prevalence. Since the 1994 ICPD, contraceptive prevalence has increased in all but two high-fertility countries (figure II.10). Countries in Eastern Africa stand out as having had dramatic increases in contraceptive prevalence such as in Ethiopia where contraceptive use increased more than tenfold from 1994 to 2014. Contraceptive prevalence remains low among high-fertility countries in Middle Africa and Western Africa even though there have been some countries in these regions with high increases in relative terms. In Gambia and Togo, contraceptive prevalence declined between 1994 and 2014. Some countries had surprisingly high levels of contraceptive prevalence, given that these are high-fertility countries. Contraceptive prevalence is above 60 per cent in Bolivia, Honduras, Jordan and Swaziland, even bearing in mind that the contraceptive use estimates refer only to married or in-union women.

Figure II.10. Contraceptive prevalence rate (CPR) in 1994 and 2014, high-fertility countries

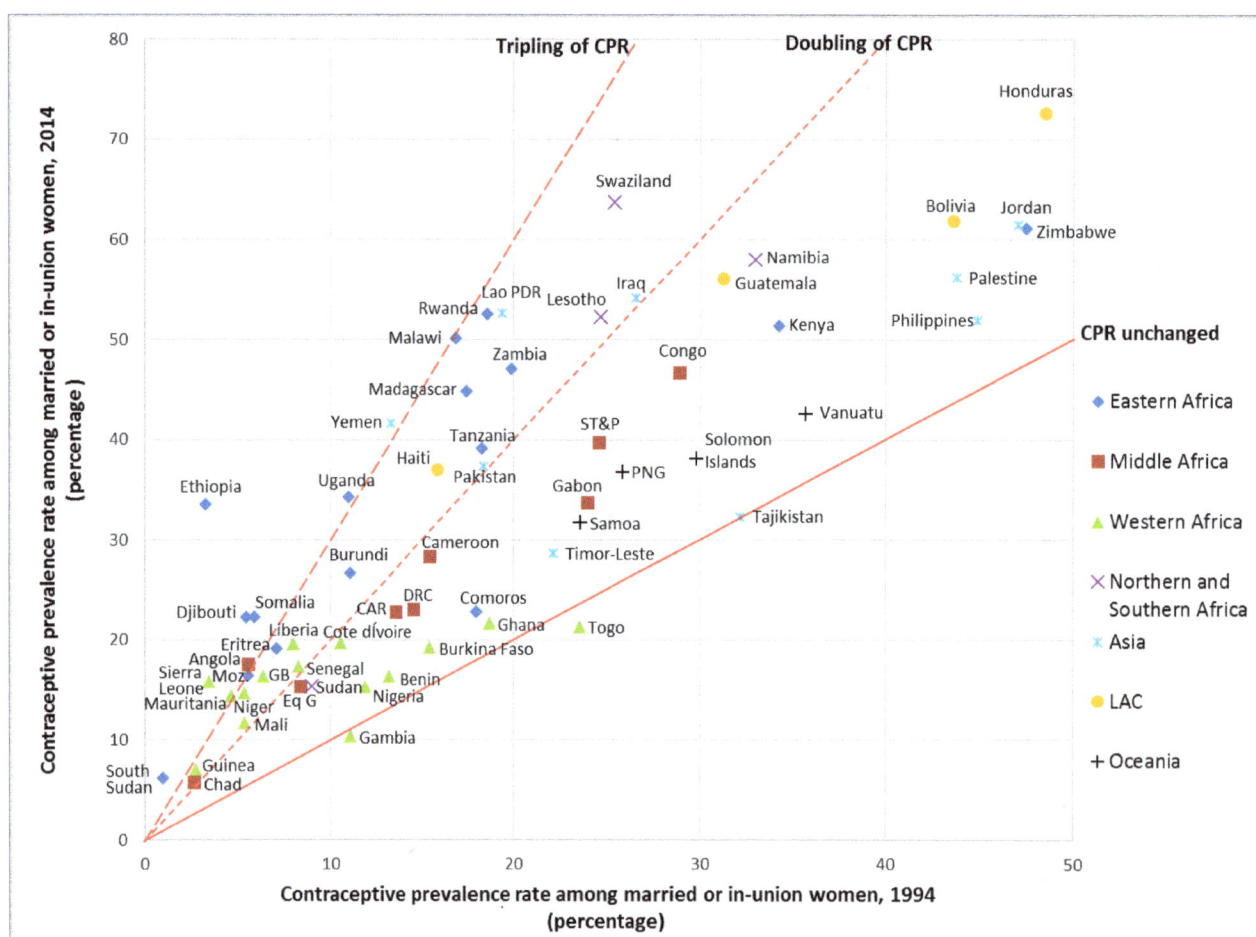

Source: United Nations 2014a.

NOTE: CAR refers to Central Africa Republic, DRC refers to Democratic Republic of Congo, Eq G refers to Equatorial Guinea, GB refers to Guinea Bissau, LAC refers to Latin America and the Caribbean, Lao PDR refers to Lao People's Democratic Republic, PNG refers to Papua New Guinea, ST&P refers to Sao Tome and Principe.

In many high-fertility countries in Middle Africa and Western Africa, the relationship between contraceptive prevalence and total fertility is weak, with fertility declining despite little increase in contraceptive prevalence (figure II.11). In most of these countries, the use of traditional methods has decreased at the same time as the use of modern methods has increased. Since modern contraceptives are usually more effective than traditional contraceptives, this can partially explain the decrease in fertility despite the limited increase in overall contraceptive use.

Many high-fertility countries in Eastern Africa show the opposite pattern where, while contraceptive use has greatly increased, the impact on total fertility has been more muted than in other high-fertility countries, although there is wide variability in the relationship between contraceptive prevalence and total fertility. In Asia and Latin American and Caribbean, there have been both sharp declines in total fertility with increases in contraceptive use, with some exceptions. Garenne (2014) points out the importance of induced abortion, and the lack of data thereof, in mitigating the relationship between trends in contraceptive use and fertility.

Figure II.11. Change in total fertility between 1990-1995 and 2005-2010 and change in contraceptive prevalence rate between 1994 and 2010, high-fertility countries

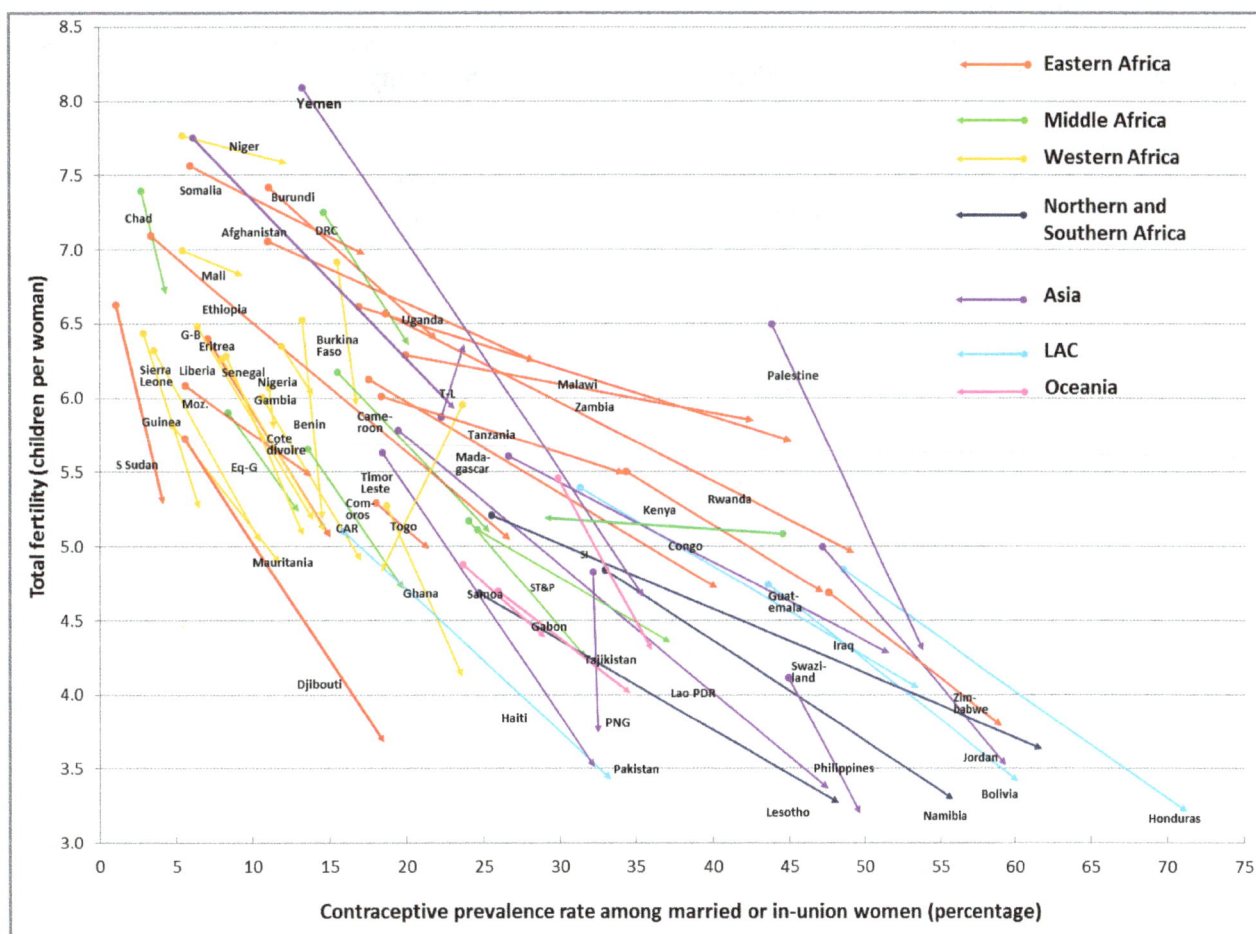

Source: United Nations (2013a) and United Nations (2014a).
NOTES: CA refers to Central African Republic, DRC refers to Democratic Republic of Congo, Eq-G refers to Equatorial Guinea, GB refers to Guinea-Bissau, LAC refers to Latin America and the Caribbean, Moz refers to Mozambique, PNG refers to Papua New Guinea, SL refers to Sierra Leone, ST&P refers to Sao Tome and Principe, TL refers to Timor-Leste.

The relationship between the change in contraceptive prevalence and change in total fertility is stronger among high-fertility countries in Asia than those in other regions. High-fertility countries in Eastern Africa, Northern Africa and Southern Africa are more similar to countries in Asia, whereas Middle African and Western African countries are more similar to Latin American and Caribbean countries where the change in total fertility is less closely associated with contraceptive use.

Contraceptive use includes many traditional methods that are generally less effective in preventing pregnancy than modern contraceptive methods. The uptake of modern methods of contraception tends to account for contemporary fertility declines more so than the use of traditional methods. An increase in contraceptive use overall without a parallel increase in the use of modern methods is unlikely to have an impact on fertility. Most high-fertility countries in Eastern Africa have seen notable gains in modern contraceptive prevalence together with declines in total fertility, although the fertility declines have been less steep than those observed in high-fertility countries in Asia and Latin America and the Caribbean.

3. *Unmet need for family planning*

In the majority of high-fertility countries, the increase in contraceptive prevalence has not kept pace with increasing demand. The percentage of women with an unmet need for family planning (i.e., women who wish to postpone their next pregnancy or stop having children altogether but, for whatever reason, are not using contraception) indicates the degree to which high-fertility countries have not addressed demand for contraceptives. Among high-fertility countries, unmet need for family planning ranges from 11 per cent of married women of reproductive age to 37 per cent (latest data point available). High-fertility countries in Asia and Latin America and the Caribbean tend to have lower levels of unmet need than countries in Eastern Africa, Middle Africa and Western Africa. However, there are some high-fertility countries in Western Africa, such as Niger and Nigeria, that also have relatively low levels of unmet need due to high desired fertility.

Unmet need can be for either limiting childbearing (when a woman wishes to have no more children) or for delaying or spacing births (when a woman wishes to have a child two or more years later). It is important to make this distinction because different types of contraception are relevant for the different types of unmet need. Among high-fertility countries with low levels of contraceptive prevalence, the vast majority of unmet need is for spacing. Most high-fertility countries with the highest percentage of unmet need for spacing are in sub-Saharan Africa, except Haiti and Timor Leste (figure II.12). Unmet need for limiting among high-fertility countries in Middle Africa and Western Africa is lower than among high-fertility countries in Asia and Latin America and the Caribbean. Although meeting unmet need for family planning is important for social and health reasons, the fertility impact of meeting unmet need for spacing is considered to be less than meeting unmet need for limiting, which partially explains a weak relationship between fertility decline and meeting demand for contraception in sub-Saharan Africa (Casterline and El-Zeini, 2014).

Figure II.12. Unmet need for limiting and for spacing, latest data available, high-fertility countries

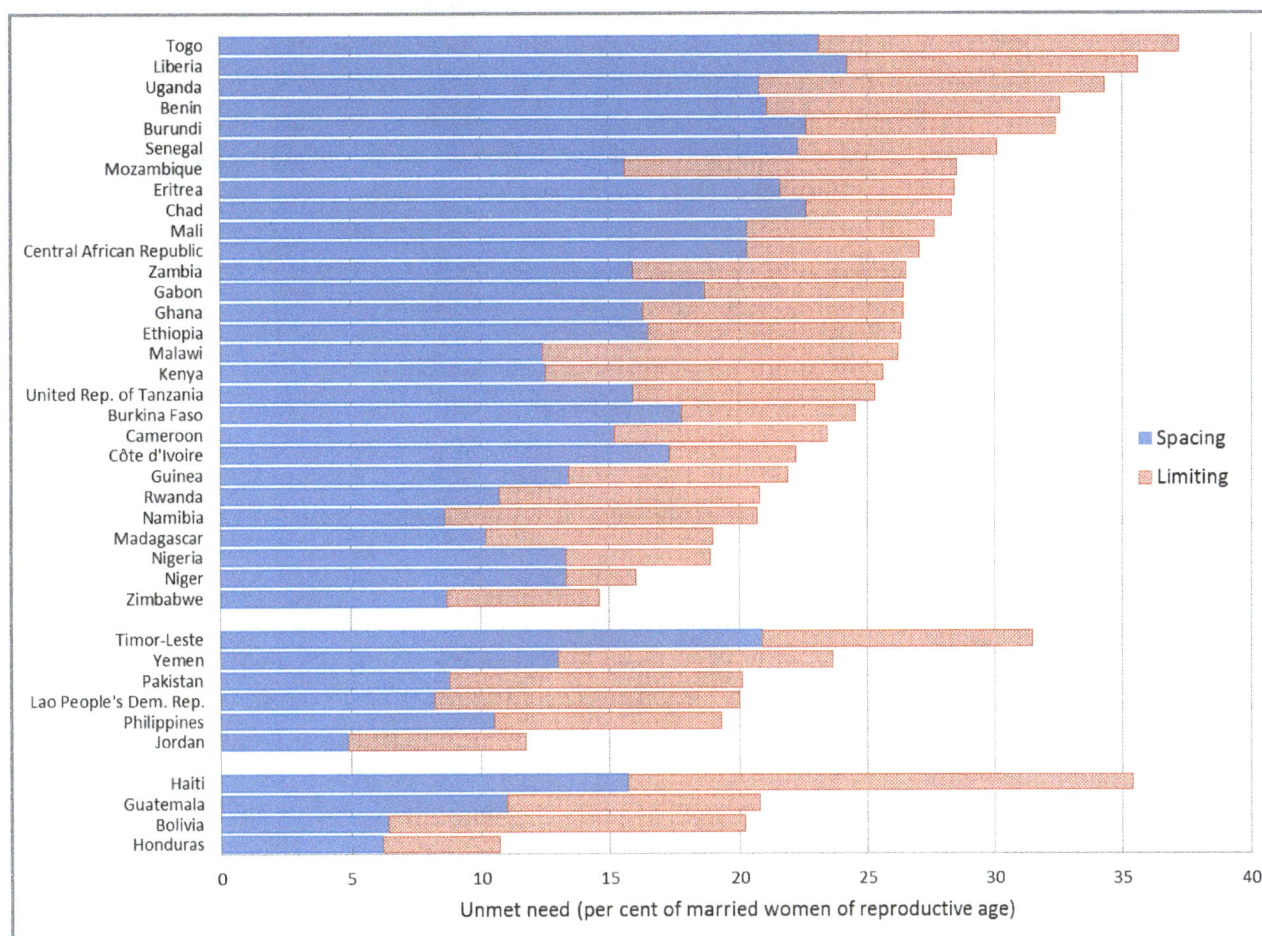

Source: United Nations (2014c).

D. FERTILITY DECLINE AND SOCIO-ECONOMIC DEVELOPMENT

The speed of the fertility transition and the timing of its onset are associated with the level of socio-economic development. Countries that have undergone recent fertility transitions have done so at increasingly lower levels of socio-economic development compared with countries where the fertility transition happened longer ago. Some of these countries have also had particularly rapid fertility declines. The experiences of countries that have undergone recent transitions to low fertility may be more informative for the future trajectory of fertility decline for today's high-fertility countries than the experiences of countries, such as countries in Europe, where fertility has been low for decades.

Two countries where fertility declined very rapidly following the onset of fertility transition are Iran and Viet Nam. Fertility levels at the onset of transition in Iran and Viet Nam were similar to those among today's high-fertility countries. In Iran, it took 25 years to move from the maximum total fertility to the level of total fertility when the fertility transition began compared to just 8 years for Viet Nam. In figures II.13 and II.14, high-fertility countries in the quartile with the longest duration (20 to 41 years) between peak and transition total fertility are compared with Iran and those in the quartile with the shortest duration (2 to 10 years) between peak and transition total fertility are compared with Viet Nam. Trend data for four socio-economic indicators are shown: the percentage of urban population, years of school life expectancy for females from primary to secondary, infant mortality rate and contraceptive prevalence. No country has attained middle-income status without urban population growth and few have reached income levels of $10,000 per capita before reaching about 60 per cent urbanization (Annez and Buckley, 2009). Urban population growth creates structural shifts that are necessary in attaining middle-income status, higher school completion rates, improved water and sanitation facilities and higher levels of contraceptive use. Research also shows that child survival and family planning programmes play important complementary roles in fertility decline (Cohen and Montgomery, 1997).

For most high-fertility countries, the fertility transition started when socio-economic indicators were at lower levels that appear insufficient to spur rapid fertility decline (as was the case for Iran and Viet Nam). Among high-fertility countries with the longest durations between peak and transition total fertility (similar to Iran's pattern), the level of urbanization tended to be lower and with somewhat slower growth over time than what occurred in Iran and the number of years of schooling from primary to secondary for girls was shorter (figure II.13). Among high-fertility countries with the shortest durations between peak and transition total fertility (similar to Viet Nam's pattern), countries tended to begin their fertility transitions at lower levels of female education but there was no clear pattern with respect to urbanization levels.

For both groups of high-fertility countries, the fertility transition began when there were higher levels of infant mortality and lower contraceptive prevalence levels compared with the low-fertility countries of Iran and Viet Nam at the time of their fertility transitions (figure II.14). For example, contraceptive prevalence at the onset of the fertility transition was 47 per cent in Iran and 29 per cent in Viet Nam, and levels rose steeply since that time point to over 75 per cent by 2010. In contrast, contraceptive prevalence was much lower at the time the fertility transition began for almost all of today's high-fertility countries and the pace of increase has been much slower.

Figure II.13 Proportion of urban population and years of school life expectancy for females among high-fertility countries in the quartiles with longest and shortest durations between the timing of peak fertility and the onset of fertility transition, high-fertility countries

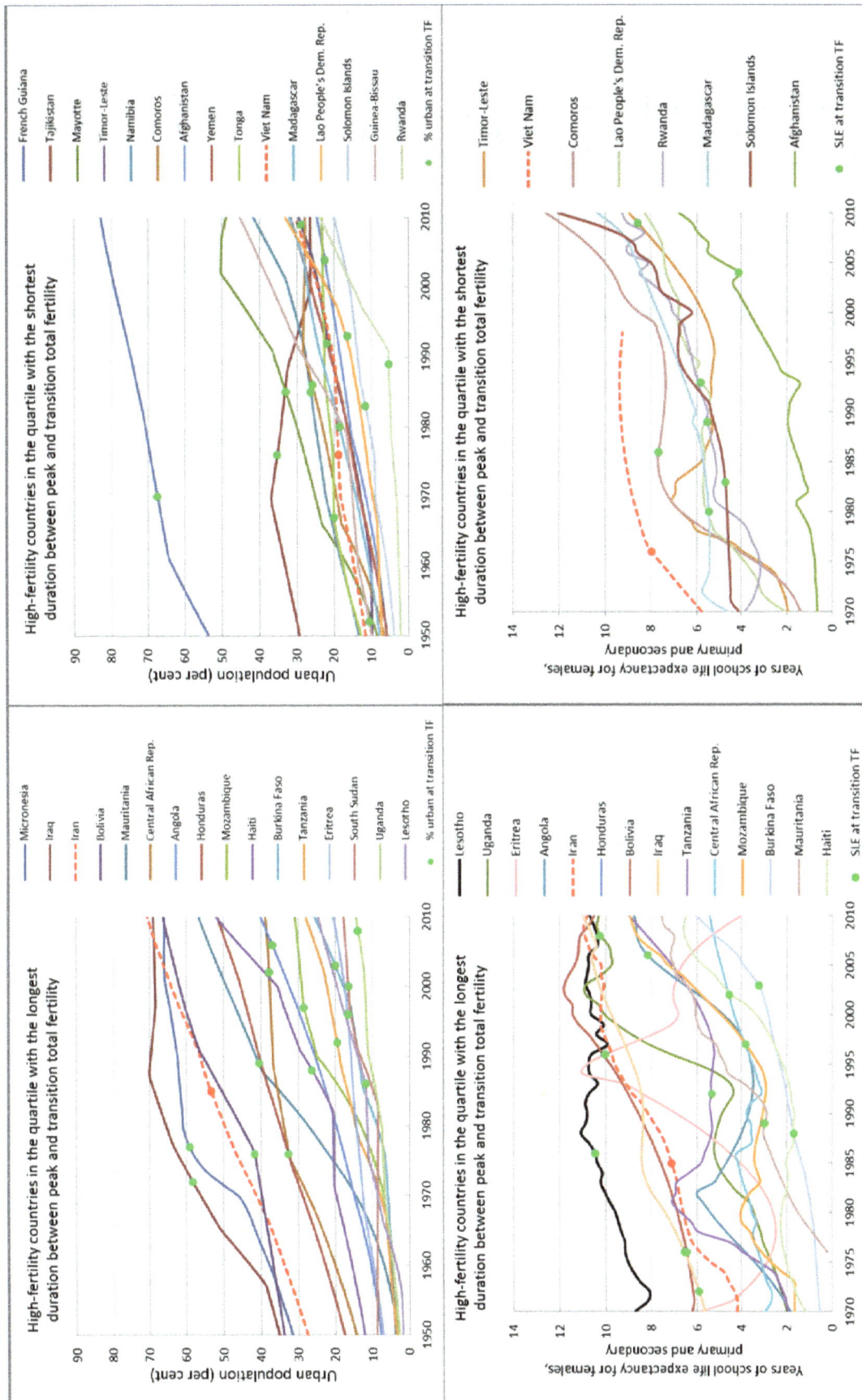

Source: UNESCO Institute for Statistics, Data Centre, 2014; United Nations (2013a, 2014d).
NOTE: SLE is school life expectancy.s

Figure II.14 Infant mortality and contraceptive prevalence among high-fertility countries in the quartiles with longest and shortest durations between the timing of peak fertility and onset of the fertility transition, high-fertility countries

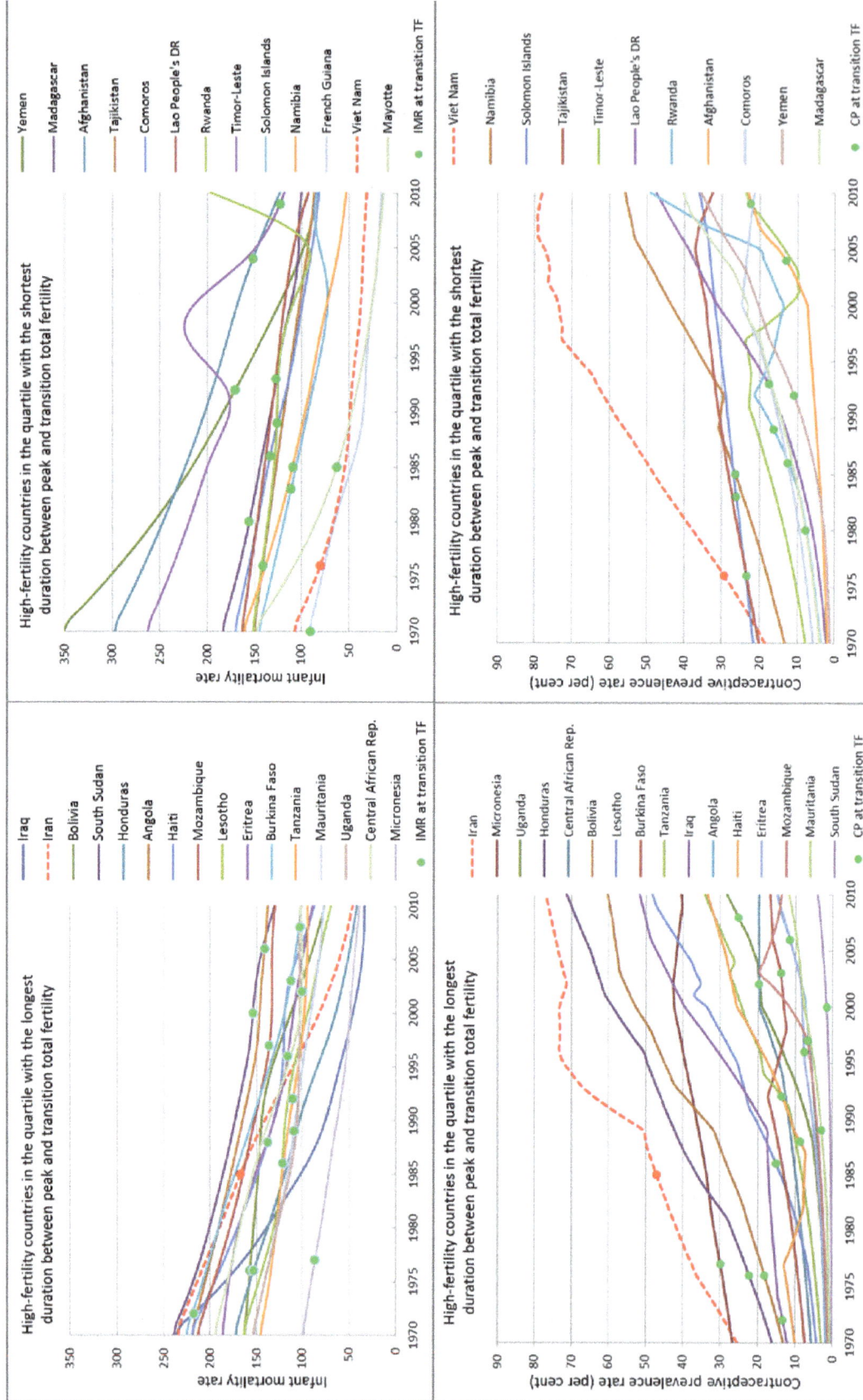

Source: United Nations (2013a, 2014a).
NOTE: IMR is infant mortality rate, CP is contraceptive prevalence.

E. Consequences of high fertility

Sustained high fertility has profound implications for population growth, the age structure, the provision of public services, maternal and child health, and the environment and natural resources. At the time of the 1994 ICPD, high fertility was common in the majority of countries in developing regions. Now, high fertility levels are predominantly in sub-Saharan Africa with only a small number of high-fertility countries outside of this region. Although there are fewer high-fertility countries today, and many have undergone significant declines in fertility, these countries will continue to contribute an increasing proportion to global population growth (Andreev and others, 2013) and the attendant development implications of a fast-growing population at the national level.

Fertility rates are the most significant driver of population age structures. Where fertility rates are high and sustained, populations will grow and have a more youthful structure. A rapid decline in fertility, where fertility rates have been high in the past, can eventually lead to a bulge in the working-age population and smaller populations of older adults and children. With such a bulge in the working-age population, it is possible to unleash enormous economic gains (May 2012:49)—the so-called "demographic dividend"—yet the gains from the demographic dividend are not an automatic result from age-structure changes. These changes can yield economic benefits if countries make investments in human capital, especially schooling, job growth and good governance, encouraging financial investment and savings (Bloom and others, 2003; Bloom and Canning, 2008; Eloundou-Enyegue, 2013).

The consequences of high fertility for education are complex. The rapid population growth that accompanies high fertility levels makes provision of public services like schooling more challenging as these services need to keep pace with the growing population. Where fertility declines rapidly, children have higher education levels, there is greater asset accumulation and greater use of preventive health services (Bongaarts and others, 2012). Evidence from Bangladesh shows that in areas experiencing lower fertility, children complete more schooling (Joshi and Schultz, 2012). The number of siblings also negatively correlates with schooling outcomes in developing countries (National Research Council and Institute of Medicine, 2005). The inverse relationship between education and fertility could also exacerbate inequalities since fertility usually decreases first among more educated mothers (Elondou-Enyegue and Williams, 2006).

Reductions in high fertility are also associated with positive trends in maternal mortality. In particular, fertility reductions generally translate into fewer risky pregnancies such as those of very young or very old mothers, those at high parity and of women with closely-spaced pregnancies (Campbell and Graham, 2006; Ahmed and others, 2012; Bongaarts and others, 2012; Cleland and others, 2012). Family planning is a key component for achieving fertility declines and reductions in maternal mortality, and it has the additional benefit of reducing the number of unintended pregnancies and therefore maternal mortality and morbidity due to unsafe abortion (Ahmed and others, 2012; Cleland and others, 2012).

The health benefits of fertility decline extend to children as well. Decreasing fertility is often associated with increasing birth intervals, especially in sub-Saharan Arica. Shorter birth intervals are known to be associated with decreased child survival: the shorter the birth interval, the greater the risk of mortality (Rutstein, 2008; Rutstein and Winter, 2014). Data show associations between birth interval length below 33 months and adverse perinatal outcomes, probably related to maternal nutritional depletion (Rutstein, 2008). For early childhood mortality, there is no threshold in the effect of interval length with the longer the interval, the smaller the risk of dying (Rutstein, 2008). The mechanisms are complicated but thought to include competition for resources and cross-infection from older siblings (Bongaarts and others, 2012). Rapid subsequent births also raise mortality for older siblings (Hobcraft and others, 1985). Since preferred birth intervals exceed three years in many sub-Saharan African countries, meeting the relatively high proportion of unmet need for family planning for spacing in these countries could improve child survival even without a change in desired family size (Bongaarts and others, 2012).

Children from high-order births (order four and higher) are known to be at greater risk of dying during childhood (Rutstein and Winter, 2014), therefore reducing unintended higher-order births through decreasing fertility will lead to decreased child mortality. In addition, similar to maternal mortality, maternal age also has an impact on child survival, with a significantly higher risk of dying throughout childhood to children born to mothers less than 18 years. For children born to older mothers over 35 years, the excess risk only exists for neonatal mortality and is balanced by a reduced risk of dying for children aged one to four years (Rutstein and Winter, 2014).

Lastly, high fertility and the high rate of population growth that it fosters can have a negative impact on the environment and natural resources (United Nations, 2011; World Bank, 2010). While there are questions over the direct relationship between demographic change and the environment, population growth has been implicated in deforestation and desertification, two outcomes that are of particular importance for poor agrarian countries, especially in sub-Saharan Africa (World Bank, 2010). Sahelian countries (Burkina Faso, Chad, Gambia, Guinea-Bissau, Mali, Mauritania, Niger and Senegal) are particularly vulnerable to the consequences of climate change and are also countries that face high population growth rates (Bongaarts and others, 2012). For example, Niger already has severe food shortages and high levels of malnutrition among children that are predicted to be exacerbated by high population growth and the expected impacts of climate change and environmental degradation, leading to greater risk of humanitarian crises in the coming decades (May, 2012, p. 163; Potts and others, 2011).

F. POLICY APPROACHES TO HIGH FERTILITY

High fertility and associated population growth present major challenges to Governments. In response to such challenges, a variety of public policies have either been considered or implemented to reduce fertility levels. High-fertility countries varied in their policy approaches towards fertility around the time of the 1994 ICPD, but many countries have since moved to adopt policies to lower fertility (figure II.15).This general change among high-fertility countries towards policies to reduce fertility is part of a longer trend reaching back to the 1970s. As of 2013, Equatorial Guinea was the only high-fertility country that remained with a policy to raise fertility.

Figure II.15. Percentage of high-fertility countries with government policies on fertility levels by type of policy, 1996 and 2013

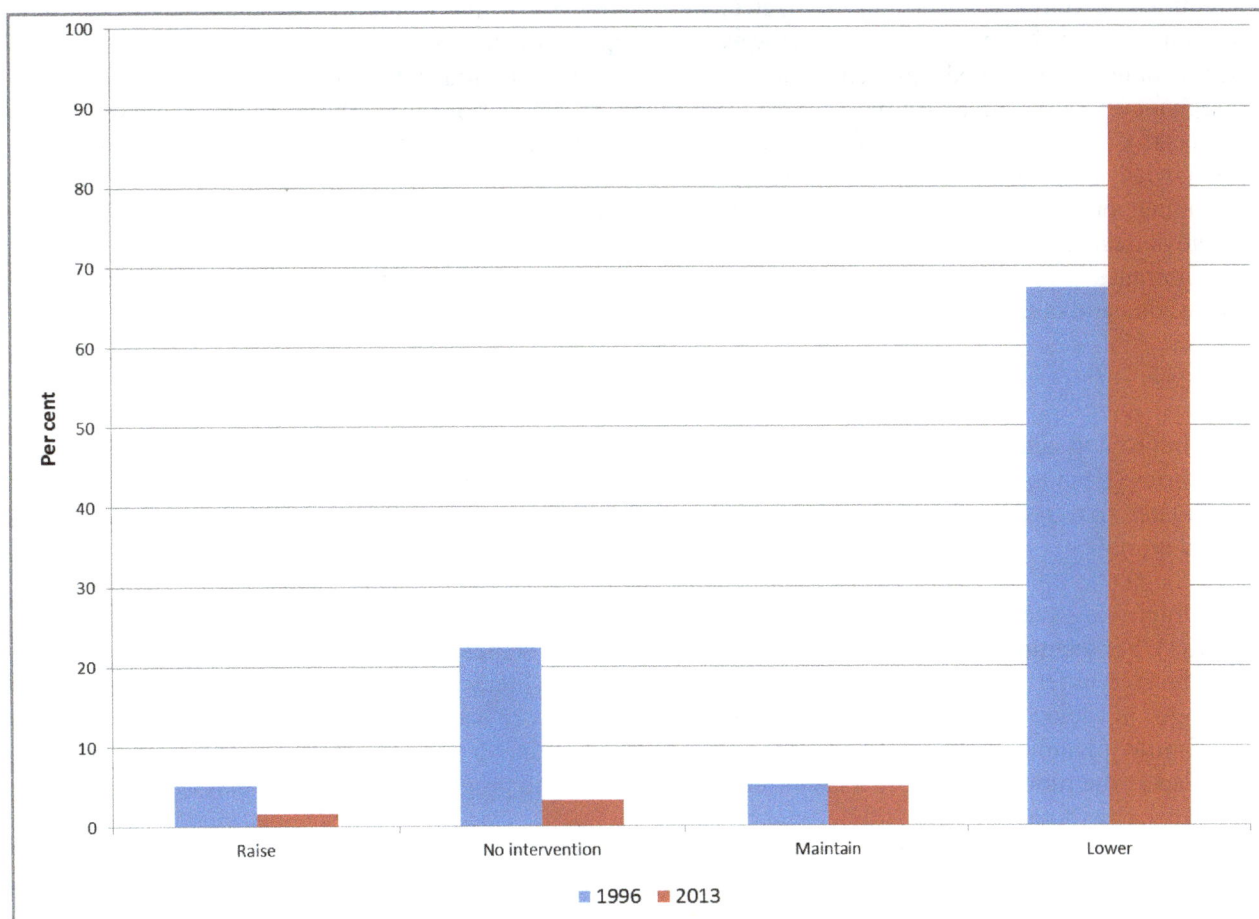

Source: United Nations (2013c).

1. *Family planning programmes*

One of the most common approaches to accelerate the reduction of fertility is to invest in high-quality, voluntary family planning programmes. Family planning is considered highly cost effective and, with sufficient political will and resources, well-run programmes have brought about sustained declines in fertility across much of Asia, the Middle East and Latin America by meeting unmet need (Bongaarts and Sinding, 2011; Kohler and Behrman, 2014; May, 2012). No country with low levels of human development has experienced deep and sustained reductions in fertility levels without a strong and committed government family planning programme. For example, the experiences of Kenya in the 1980s and Rwanda in recent years shows that strong Government-led efforts can be as effective in Africa as they were in Asia and elsewhere three decades ago (Bongaarts and others, 2012; May, 2012).

The rapid declines in fertility in Asia and Latin America and the Caribbean were mainly due to the realization of existing demand for smaller families, but in high-fertility countries today there needs to be a change in the demand for children to achieve similar declines (World Bank, 2010). Evidence suggests that family planning programmes can also have an influence on the desired family sizes and fertility preferences (Bongaarts, 2011; Das Gupta and others, 2011; Westoff, 2012).

Family planning programmes can also address barriers to use that go beyond basic supply challenges. For example, Uganda has much higher fertility and lower contraceptive use than in the neighbouring countries of Kenya, Rwanda and Zimbabwe, and yet two out of five young women aged 15-24 years have an unmet need for family planning. However, multiple obstacles, including strong misconceptions and fears about using methods, prevent young women from using contraception despite their desire to prevent pregnancy (Nalwadda and others, 2010). Improving dissemination of information about contraception, especially through media, and with a particular focus on vulnerable groups of people such as the young, unmarried, poor and rural (Darroch, 2013; Das Gupta and others, 2011) should be priorities of family planning programmes. Given the inequities in reproductive decision-making power to women's disadvantage in many high-fertility countries, it may be more effective to integrate family planning programmes with other strategies that promote gender-equitable norms (Izugbara and Ezeh, 2010; Nalwadda and others, 2010).

2. *Education and other approaches that influence fertility decline*

Improving access to female education is imperative to a sustained fertility transition in high-fertility countries (Ezeh and others, 2009; Lutz, 2014), both as a factor on its own and also due to its association with later marriage, the demand for and ability to obtain and use contraceptives, and declines in infant and child mortality (Lutz, 2014; Shapiro and Gebreselassie, 2008).

Improving socioeconomic conditions are also associated with continued fertility decline (May, 2012, p. 131). For example, in Kenya, low and deteriorating living standards are thought to be partly responsible for the stall in fertility decline, despite high levels of female literacy and schooling (Bongaarts, 2006) and changes in socioeconomic conditions in Ghana have been more decisive for fertility decline than changes in family planning services (Agyei-Mensah, 2006). Similarly, socioeconomic interventions are also needed as the rural poor are often resentful of family planning programmes that they may not identify as a high priority (Agei-Mensah, 2006).

In countries where large proportions of girls still marry before the age of 18 years, policies and programmes promoting a later age at marriage can be effective in reducing early childbearing (National Research Council and Institute of Medicine, 2005). In the Berhane Hewan Programme in Ethiopia, for example, economic incentives were provided to families who did not marry off their daughters during the project period and support was provided for girls who were already married (Erulkar and Muthengi, 2009). Adolescent girls in the experimental area were nearly three times more likely to be in school, were 90 per cent less likely to be married and were nearly three times more likely to have used any family planning method compared to girls in the control area (Erulkar and Muthengi, 2009).

Declining infant and child mortality are also argued to be a pre-requisite for fertility decline and future fertility changes are dependent on the future of changes in infant and child mortality (Shapiro and Gebreselassie, 2008). While improvements in child survival are essential, increases in child survival in most high-fertility African countries have already exceeded the level at which steep fertility declines began in many countries of other regions (Bongaarts and others, 2012).

3. *The distinctiveness of sub-Saharan Africa*

The pace of future fertility decline for high-fertility countries today, most of which are in sub-Saharan Africa, may be distinctly different than in other regions (Bongaarts 2013; Bongaarts and Casterline, 2012). For example, meeting unmet need for family planning has less of an impact on fertility in this region (Casterline and El-Zeini, 2014), with women often postponing births in order to space rather than limit family size (Moultrie and others, 2012; Romaniuk, 2011). The onset of the fertility transition also took place at generally lower levels of development than was the case for countries that have more recently made the transition from high fertility to low fertility. This variance from historical patterns is important not only for planning and implementing policies that may reduce fertility, but also because it may have far-reaching development implications.

CONCLUSION

Fertility levels have undergone remarkable changes throughout the world since the 1994 International Conference on Population and Development. This report focused on fertility and its correlates at the extremes: countries with very low fertility and those with very high fertility. High fertility is increasingly a characteristic of the least developed countries, especially in sub-Saharan Africa. Low fertility, previously a characteristic of countries in Europe, has become far more widespread in other regions, with some countries experiencing very rapid fertility transitions at lower levels of human development than was the case historically.

Considerable diversity exists at the extremes in terms of the pathways that resulted in low or high fertility and the factors underlying fertility change, even among countries with similar fertility levels. This raises questions about the future course that fertility will take. The fertility transition in countries in sub-Saharan Africa has been exceptional in that it has been slower, later, and at a lower level of development than countries in Asia and Latin America and the Caribbean (Bongaarts, 2013). As a result, it has been suggested that the pace of fertility decline in sub-Saharan Africa has been projected to be too rapid (United Nations, 2013e), especially outside of Southern Africa. Others argue that gains in women's education in these countries will help usher in faster fertility declines than initially projected (Lutz and others, 2014). Similarly, many questions remain regarding the fertility projections for low-fertility countries. There is no evidence that the recent increase in period fertility levels in some European countries will be emulated by countries in other regions with very low fertility, such as Eastern Asia.

The age pattern of childbearing is important for fertility trends since changes in the age of childbearing can have a significant impact on both period and completed fertility as well as implications for maternal and infant health. There have been significant declines in adolescent childbearing in high-fertility countries, although the rates remain high in Middle Africa and Western Africa. In the majority of high-fertility countries, the decline in fertility among older women contributed a large proportion of the overall decline in total fertility since the ICPD rather than the decline in adolescent fertility. At the other extreme, childbearing among older women is becoming more prevalent in low-fertility countries. In Latin America and the Caribbean, childbearing at young ages remains relatively high despite the decline in total fertility to low levels.

Government policies to influence fertility, whether to raise or lower it, have changed significantly since the ICPD in 1994. There is now far more concern about fertility levels, with more low-fertility countries expressing concern about and adopting policies to raise fertility and high-fertility countries doing the same to lower fertility. For some countries, the change in policy came about due to a realisation of the impact of continued fertility levels at either the high or low extremes. In other countries, in particular the low-fertility countries that had very rapid fertility transitions, policies changed to accommodate a new demographic reality. While demography is not destiny, the implications of fertility levels at the extremes will continue to reflect and shape the well-being of individuals, families, countries and, ultimately, the world.

REFERENCES

Abbasi-Shavazi, Mohammad Jalal, and Bhakta Gubhaju (2014). Different pathways to low fertility in Asia: Consequences and Policy Implications. Expert Paper No. 2014/1. New York: United Nations. Available from http://www.un.org/en/development/desa/population/publications/pdf/expert/2014-1_Abbasi-Shavazi&GubhajuExpert-Paper.pdf.

Agyei-Mensah, Samuel (2006). Fertility transition in Ghana: Looking back and looking forward. *Population, Space and Place*, No. 12, pp. 461-477.

Ahmed, Saifuddin, Qingfeng Li, Li Liu and Amy O. Tsui (2012). Maternal deaths averted by contraceptive use: An analysis of 172 countries. *The Lancet*, vol. 380, No. 9837, pp. 111-125.

Andersson, Gunnar (2008). A review of policies and practices related to the 'Highest-Low' fertility of Sweden. *Vienna Yearbook of Population Research*, pp. 89-102.

Andreev, Kirill, Vladimíra Kantorová and John Bongaarts (2013). Demographic components of future population growth. Technical Paper No. 2013/3. New York: United Nations. Available from http://www.un.org/en/development/desa/population/publications/pdf/technical/TP2013-3.pdf.

Annez, Patricia Clarke and Robert M. Buckley (2009). Urbanization and growth: Setting the context. In *Urbanization and Growth: Commission on Growth and Development*, Spence M, Annez P C, and Buckley R M, eds. Washington, DC. The International Bank for Reconstruction and Development . The World Bank, pp.1–46.

Balbo, Nicoletta, Francesco Billari, and Melinda Mills (2013). Fertility in advanced societies: A review of research. *European Journal of Population*, vol. 29, pp. 1-38.

Berent, Jerzy (1970). Causes of fertility decline in Eastern Europe and the Soviet Union: Part I. The influence of demographic factors. *Population Studies*, vol. 24, No. 1, pp. 35–58.

Billingsley, Sunnee and Tommy Ferrarini (2014). Family policy and fertility intentions in 21 European countries. *Journal of Marriage and Family*, vol. 76, pp. 428-445.

Blanc, Ann, William Winfrey and John Ross (2013). New findings for maternal mortality age patterns: Aggregated results for 38 countries. *PLoS ONE*, vol. 8, No. 4, e59864. Available from http://www.ploscollections.org/article/info%3Adoi%2F10.1371%2Fjournal.pone.0059864.

Bloom, David E. and David Canning (2008) Global demographic change: Dimensions and economic significance. *Population and Development Review,* vol. 34(S), pp.17-51.

Bloom, David E., David Canning, and Jaypee Sevilla (2003). *The Demographic Dividend: A New Perspective on the Economic Consequences of Population Change.* RAND Corporation, Monograph Reports MR-1274-WFHF/DLPF/RF/UNPF.

Boling, P. (2008). Demography, culture and policy: Understanding Japan's low fertility. *Population and Development Review*, vol. 34, No. 2, pp. 307-326.

Bongaarts, John (2006). The causes of stalling fertility transitions. *Studies in Family Planning,* vol. 37, No. 1, pp. 1-16.

———— (2011). Can family planning programs reduce high desired family size in sub-Saharan Africa? *International Perspectives on Sexual and Reproductive Health*, vol. 37, No. 4, pp. 209-216.

———— (2013). How exceptional is the pattern of fertility decline in sub-Saharan Africa? Expert Paper No. 2013/4. New York: United Nations. Available from http://www.un.org/en/development/desa/population/publications/pdf/expert/2013-4_Bongaarts_Expert-Paper.pdf.

Bongaarts, John, and John Casterline (2012). Fertility transition: Is sub-Saharan Africa different? *Population and Development Review*, vol. 38 (Supplement s1), pp. 153-168.

Bongaarts, John, John Cleland, John Townsend, Jane Bertrand, and Monica Das Gupta (2012). *Family Planning Programs for the 21st Century Rationale and Design*. New York, NY: Population Council.

Bongaarts, John, and Steven Sinding (2011). Population policy in transition in the developing world. *Science* , vol. 333, pp. 574-576.

Campbell, Oona, and Wendy Graham (2006). Strategies for reducing maternal mortality: Getting on with what works. *The Lancet* , vol. 368, pp. 1284-1299.

Casterline, John and El-Zeini, Laila (2014). Unmet need and fertility decline: A comparative perspective on prospects in sub-Saharan Africa. *Studies in Family Planning,* vol. 45, No. 2, pp. 227-245.

Cavenaghi, Suzana. 2013. Fertility decline and public policies to address population rights: Perspective from Latin America. Expert Paper No. 2013/5. New York: United Nations. Available from http://www.un.org/en/development/desa/population/publications/pdf/expert/2013-5_Cavenaghi_ Expert-Paper.pdf.

Cleland, John, Agustin Conde-Agudelo, Herbert Peterson, John Ross and Amy Tsui (2012). Contraception and health. *The Lancet*, vol. 380, No. 9837, pp. 149-156.

Coale, Ansley (1986). The decline of fertility in Europe since the eighteenth century as a chapter in demographic history. In *The Decline of Fertility in Europe* , Coale A and Watkins S, eds. Princeton: Princeton University Press, pp.1-30.

Cohen, Barney and Mark R. Montgomery (1997). Introduction. In *From Death to Birth: Mortality Decline and Reproductive Change*, Cohen B and Montgomery M R, eds. Washington, DC, Committee on Population, National Research Council, pp.1–38.

Darroch, Jacqueline E. (2013). Trends in contraceptive use. *Contraception*, vol. 87, pp. 259-263.

Das Gupta, Monica, John Bongaarts, and John Cleland (2011). Population, poverty, and sustainable development: A review of the evidence. The World Bank Development Research Group, Policy Research Working Paper 5719.

Duvander, Ann-Zofie, Trude Lappegård, and Gunnar Andersson (2010). Family policy and fertility: Fathers' and mothers' use of parental leave and continued childbearing in Norway and Sweden. *Journal of European Social Policy,* vol. 20, No. 1, pp. 19-31.

Eloundou-Enyegue, Parfait (2013). Harnessing a demographic dividend: Challenges and opportunities in high and intermediate fertility countries. Expert Paper No. 2013/7. New York: United Nations. Available from http://www.un.org/en/development/desa/population/publications/pdf/expert/2013-7_Eloundou-EnyegueExpert-Paper.pdf.

Eloundou-Enyegue, Parfait and Linda Williams (2006). Family size and schooling in sub-Saharan African settings: A reexamination. *Demography*, vol. 43, No. 1, pp. 25-52.

Erulkar, Annabel and Eunice Muthengi (2009). *Evaluation of Berhane Hewan: A Pilot Program to Promote Education & Delay Marriage in Rural Ethiopia*. New York: The Population Council.

Ezeh, Alex, John Bongaarts, and Blessing Mberu. (2012). Global population trends and policy options. *The Lancet*, vol. 380, No. 9837, pp. 142-148.

Ezeh, Alex, Blessing Mberu, and Jacques Emina (2009). Stall in fertility decline in Eastern African countries: Regional analysis of patterns, determinants and implications. *Philosophical Transactions of the Royal Society B: Biological Sciences, vol.* 364, pp. 2991-3007.

Frejka, T., G. W. Jones, and J.P. Sardon. (2010) East Asian childbearing patterns and policy developments. *Population and Development Review*, vol. 36, pp. 579–606.

Garenne, Michel (2014) Trends in marriage and contraception in sub-Saharan Africa: A longitudinal perspective on factors of fertility decline. DHS Analytical Studies No. 42. ICF International Rockville, Maryland.

Gauthier. A. H. (2007). The impact of family policies on fertility in industrialized countries: A review of the literature. *Population Research and Policy* Review, vol. 26, No. 3, pp. 323-346.

——— (2008). Some theoretical and methodological comments on the impact of policies on fertility. *Vienna Yearbook of Population Research*, pp. 25-28.

Gauthier, A. H., and D. Philipov (2008). Can policies enhance fertility in Europe? *Vienna Yearbook of Population Research*, pp. 1-16.

Guo, Zhigang (2012). The low fertility rate is the major demographic risk in China. *China Economic Journal*, vol. 5, pp. 2-3.

Hobcraft, J.N., J.W. McDonald, and S.O. Rutstein (1985). Demographic determinants of infant and early child mortality: A comparative analysis. *Demography*, vol. 39, No. 3, pp. 363-385.

Hoorens, Stijn, Jack Clift, Laura Staetsky, Barbara Janta, Stephanie Diepeveen, Molly Morgan Jones, and Jonathan Grant (2011). *Low Fertility in Europe. Is There Still Reason to Worry?* Rand Europe. Cambridge, UK.

Izugbara, C. O. and Ezeh, A. C. (2010), Women and high fertility in Islamic Northern Nigeria. *Studies in Family Planning*, vol. 4, pp. 193–204.

Jones, Gavin (2007). Delayed marriage and very low fertility in Pacific Asia. *Population and Development Review*, vol. 33, No. 3, pp. 453-478.

——— (2010). Changing marriage patterns in Asia. Asia Research Institute Working Paper Series No. 131 Available from http://www.ari.nus.edu.sg/docs/wps/wps10_131.pdf.

——— (2012). Population policy in a prosperous city-state: Dilemmas for Singapore. *Population and Development Review*, vol. 38, pp. 311–336.

Joshi, Shareen, and T. Paul Schultz (2012). Family planning and women's and children's health: Long-term consequences of an outreach program in Matlab, Bangladesh. *Demography*, vol. 50, pp. 149-180.

Kalwij, Adriaan. 2010. The impact of family policy expenditure on fertility in Western Europe. *Demography*, vol. 47, No. 2, pp. 503-519.

Kocourkova, Jirina, Boris Burcin and Tomas Kucera (2014). Demographic relevancy of increased use of assisted reproduction in European countries. *Reproductive Health*, vol. 11, No. 37. Available from http://www.reproductive-health-journal.com/content/11/1/37.

Kohler, Hans-Peter and Jere R. Behrman (2014). Benefits and costs of the population and demography targets for the post-2015 development agenda. Copenhagen Consensus Assessment Paper. Available from http://www.copenhagenconsensus.com/post-2015-consensus/populationanddemography.

Kohler, Hans-Peter, Francesco C. Billari and José Antonio Ortega (2002). The emergence of lowest-low fertility in Europe during the 1990s. *Population and Development Review*, vol. 28, No. 4, pp. 641–680.

——— (2006). Low fertility in Europe: Causes, implications and policy options. In *The Baby Bust. Who will do the Work? Who Will Pay the Taxes?* Fred R. Harris, ed. Lanham, MD Rowman and Littlefield Publishers, pp. 48-109.

Kupka, M.S. and others (2014). Assisted reproductive technology in Europe, 2010: results generated from European registers by European Society of Human Reproduction and Embryology (ESHRE). *Human Reproduction*, vol. 29, No. 10, pp. 2099–2113.

Luci-Greulich, Angela and Olivier Thévenon (2013). The impact of family policies on fertility trends in developed countries. *European Journal of Population,* vol. 29, No. 4, pp. 387-416.

Lutz, Wolfgang (2014). A population policy rationale for the twenty-first century. *Population and Development Review*, vol. 40, No. 3, pp. 527-544.

Lutz, Wolfgang, William P. Butz and Samir KC, eds. (2014). *World Population & Human Capital in the 21st Century*. Oxford: Oxford University Press.

May, John (2012). *World Population Policies: Their Origin, Evolution, and Impact*. Springer Press, New York, USA.

Moultrie, Tom, Takudzwa Sayi, and Ian Timaeus. (2012). Birth intervals, postponement, and fertility decline in Africa: A new type of transition? *Population Studies*, vol. 66, No. 3, pp. 241-258.

Nalwadda, Gorrette, Florence Mirembe, Josaphat Byamugisha, and Elisabeth Faxelid (2010). Persistent high fertility in Uganda: Young people recount obstacles and enabling factors to use of contraceptives. *BMC Public Health*, vol. 10, No. 530, pp. 1-13.

National Research Council and Institute of Medicine (2005). *Growing Up Global: The Changing Transitions to Adulthood in Developing Countries*. Washington, D.C., The National Academies Press.

Potts, Malcolm, Virginia Gidi, Martha Campbell and Sarah Zureick (2011). Niger: Too little, too late. *International Perspectives on Sexual and Reproductive Health*, vol. 37, No. 2, pp. 95-101.

Rodríguez-Vignoli, Jorge and Suzana Cavenaghi (2014). Adolescent and youth fertility and social inequality in Latin America and the Caribbean: what role has education played? *Genus*, vol. 70, No. 1, pp. 1-25.

Romaniuk, Anatole (2011). Persistence of high fertility in Tropical Africa: The case of the Democratic Republic of the Congo. *Population and Development Review*, vol. 37, No. 1, pp. 1-28.

Rutstein, Shea (2008). Further evidence of the effects of preceding birth intervals on neonatal, infant and under-five-years mortality and nutritional status in developing countries: Evidence from the demographic and health. Calverton, MD: ORC Macro, DHS Working Paper 41. Available from http://www.dhsprogram.com/pubs/pdf/WP41/WP41.pdf

Rutstein, Shea and Rebecca Winter (2014). The effects of fertility behavior on child survival and child nutritional status: Evidence from the Demographic and Health Surveys, 2006 to 2012. DHS Analytical Studies, No. 37. ICF International Rockville, Maryland. Available from http://www.dhsprogram.com/pubs/pdf/AS37/AS37.pdf

Shapiro, David and Tesfayi Gebreselassie. (2008) Fertility transition in sub-Saharan Africa: Falling and stalling. *African Population Studies*, vol. 23, No. 1, pp. 3-23.

Sneeringer, Stacey (2009). Fertility transition in sub-Saharan Africa: Comparative analysis of cohort trends in 30 countries. DHS Comparative Reports No. 23. Calverton, MD. Available from http://dhsprogram.com/pubs/pdf/CR23/CR23.pdf.

Sobotka, Tomas. 2013. Pathways to low fertility: European perspectives. Expert Paper No. 2013/8. New York: United Nations. Available from http://www.un.org/en/development/desa/population /publications/pdf/expert/2013-8_Sobotka_Expert-Paper.pdf.

Sobotka, Tomas and Eva Beaujouan. 2014. Two is best? The persistence of a two-child family ideal in Europe. *Population and Development Review*, vol. 40, No. 3, pp. 391-419.

Stephen, Elizabeth Hervey (2012). Bracing for low fertility and a large elderly population in South Korea. Korea Economic Institute Academic Paper Series. Available from http://www.keia.org/sites/ default/files/publications/aps_doc_elizabeth_stephens.pdf.

Thévenon, Olivier (2011). Family policies in OECD countries: A comparative analysis. *Population and Development Review*, vol. 37, pp. 57–87.

Thévenon, Olivier and Anne H. Gauthier (2011). Family Policies in Developed Countries: A 'Fertility-Booster' with Side-Effects. *Community, Work & Family* vol. 14, No. 2, pp. 197-216.

United Nations (1966). World population prospects, as assessed in 1963. *Population Studies* No. 41. New York, United Nations.

United Nations, Department of Economic and Social Affairs, Population Division (2011). Seven Billion and Growing: The Role of Population Policy in Achieving Sustainability. Technical Paper No. 2011/3. New York, United Nations. Available from http://www.un.org/en/development/desa/ population/publications/pdf/technical/TP2011-3_SevenBillionandGrowing.pdf.

———— (2013a). *World Population Prospects: The 2012 Revision*. New York, United Nations. Available from http://esa.un.org/unpd/wpp/index.htm.

———— (2013b). *World Marriage Data 2012*. New York, United Nations. Available from http://www.un.org/en/development/desa/population/publications/dataset/marriage/wmd2012.shtml

———— (2013c). *World Population Policies 2013*. New York, United Nations. Available from http://www.un.org/en/development/desa/population/publications/pdf/policy/WPP2013/wpp2013.pdf .

———— (2013d). *Adolescent Fertility since the International Conference on Population and Development (ICPD) in Cairo*. New York: United Nations. Available from http://www.un.org/en/development/desa/population/publications/pdf/fertility/Report_Adolescent-Fertility-since-ICPD.pdf.

———— (2013e). *United Nations Expert Group Meeting on Fertility, Changing Population Trends and Development: Challenges and Opportunities for the Future*. New York, United Nations. Available from http://www.un.org/en/development/desa/population/events/expert-group/21/index.shtml.

———— (2014a). *Model-based Estimates and Projections of Family Planning Indicators 2014*. Available from: http://www.un.org/en/development/desa/population/theme/family-planning/cp_ model.shtml

———— (2014b). *World Population Prospects The 2012 Revision*. Methodology of the United Nations Population Estimates and Projections. New York, United Nations. Available from http://esa.un.org/unpd/wpp/Documentation/pdf/WPP2012_Methodology.pdf

———— (2014c). *World Contraceptive Use 2014* (POP/DB/CP/Rev2014). Available from http://www.un.org/en/development/desa/population/publications/dataset/contraception/wcu2014.shtml

———— (2014). *World Urbanization Prospects: The 2014 Revision*, CD-ROM Edition. New York, United Nations.

UNESCO Institute for Statistics, Data Centre (2014). Available from http://data.uis.unesco.org /Index.aspx?DataSetCode=EDULIT_DS&popupcustomise=true&lang=en (accessed 13 October 2014).

Westoff, Charles. (2012). The recent fertility transition in Rwanda. *Population and Development Review*, vol. 38 (Supplement), pp. 169-178.

Wilson, Chris, Tomáš Sobotka, Lee Williamson and Paul Boyle (2013). Migration and intergenerational replacement in Europe. *Population and Development Review*, vol. 39, No. 1, pp. 131-157.

World Bank. (2010). *Determinants and consequences of high fertility: A synopsis of the evidence.* Washington, DC: World Bank. Available from http://siteresources.worldbank.org/INTPRH/ Resources/376374-1278599377733/Determinant62810PRINT.pdf.

Annexes

Indicator	Source
Total fertility	World Population Prospects: The 2012 Revision (United Nations, 2013a)
Age-specific fertility rates	
Mean age at first birth	National sources – annex table 2 (low-fertility countries) and annex table 7 (low-fertility countries)
Completed fertility	National sources – annex table 3
Extra-marital births	National sources – annex table 4
Mean age at first marriage	National sources – annex table 7
Singulate mean age at marriage	World Marriage Data 2012 (United Nations, 2013b)
Contraceptive prevalence rate	Model-based Estimates and Projections of Family Planning Indicators 2014 (United Nations, 2014a)
Unmet need for family planning	
Fertility policies	World Population Policies 2013 (United Nations, 2013c)

Country	Year	Age	Source*	Year	Age	Source*
Armenia	1995	22.5	UNECE	2011	23.5	UNECE
Australia	1995	28.6	National statistics	2006	30.5	National statistics
Austria	1995	25.6	UNECE	2010	28.2	HFD
Azerbaijan......................	1995	23.8	UNECE	2011	23.4	UNECE
Belarus..........................	1995	22.9	UNECE	2011	25.1	UNECE
Belgium	1995	27.5	UNECE	2010	28.0	UNECE
Bosnia and Herzegovina .	1990	23.5	UNECE	2011	26.3	UNECE
Bulgaria	1995	22.2	UNECE	2011	26.6	UNECE
Canada...........................	1995	26.4	UNECE	2011	28.1	UNECE
Chile	1993	23.4	National statistics	2004	23.7	National statistics
China, Hong Kong SAR .	1996	28.8	National statistics	2008	29.8	National statistics
Croatia	1995	25.0	UNECE	2011	27.9	UNECE
Cyprus............................	1995	25.5	UNECE	2010	28.5	UNECE
Czech Republic..............	1995	22.9	UNECE	2011	27.8	HFD
Denmark	1995	27.4	UNECE	2012	29.1	UNECE
Estonia...........................	1995	23.0	UNECE	2011	26.4	HFD
Finland...........................	1995	27.2	UNECE	2012	28.5	HFD
France	1995	28.1	UNECE	2010	28.1	UNECE
Georgia	1995	23.5	UNECE	2011	24.0	UNECE
Germany	1995	28.1	UNECE	2012	29.2	UNECE
Greece............................	1995	26.6	UNECE	2010	31.2	UNECE
Hungary	1995	23.4	UNECE	2011	28.3	UNECE
Ireland............................	1995	27.0	UNECE	2012	29.9	UNECE
Italy...............................	1995	28.0	UNECE	2011	30.3	UNECE
Japan..............................	1995	27.5	National statistics	2010	29.9	National statistics
Latvia.............................	1995	23.5	UNECE	2011	26.4	UNECE
Lithuania........................	1995	23.2	UNECE	2011	26.7	HFD
Luxembourg....................	1995	27.9	UNECE	2012	30.2	UNECE
Malta..............................	1995	25.8	UNECE	2010	26.9	UNECE
Montenegro.....................	2000	25.6	UNECE	2010	26.3	UNECE
Netherlands.....................	1995	28.4	UNECE	2011	29.4	HFD
Norway	1995	26.5	UNECE	2012	28.5	UNECE
Poland............................	1995	23.8	UNECE	2011	26.9	UNECE
Portugal..........................	1995	25.8	UNECE	2012	29.5	UNECE
Republic of Korea...........	1998	27.1	National statistics	2009	29.9	National statistics
Republic of Moldova......	1995	22.0	UNECE	2011	23.7	UNECE
Romania..........................	1995	22.7	UNECE	2011	26.0	UNECE
Russian Federation..........	1995	22.6	UNECE	2010	24.9	HFD
Serbia.............................	1995	24.3	UNECE	2011	27.5	UNECE
Singapore........................	1998	28.6	National statistics	2010	29.8	National statistics
Slovakia..........................	1995	21.8	UNECE	2011	27.8	HFD
Slovenia..........................	1995	25.1	UNECE	2011	28.8	HFD
Spain..............................	1995	28.4	UNECE	2010	29.8	UNECE
Sweden	1995	27.2	UNECE	2010	28.9	HFD
Switzerland.....................	1995	28.1	UNECE	2012	30.4	HFD
TFYR Macedonia	1995	23.5	UNECE	2010	26.2	UNECE
Ukraine	1990	22.7	UNECE	2008	25.8	UNECE
United Kingdom	1994	26.5	National statistics	2012	28.1	National statistics
Viet Nam	1997	22.6	DHS 1997 (survey)	2002	22.6	DHS 2002 (survey)

NOTE: DHS is Demographic and Health Surveys, MICS is Multiple Indicator Cluster Survey, HFD is the Human Fertility Database (a joint project of the Max Planck Institute for Demographic Research and the Vienna Institute of Demography), UNECE is United Nations Economic Commission for Europe.

*Registration data unless otherwise noted.

Country	Childless			Three of more children		
	Year	Percentage	Source (data type)	Year	Percentage	Source (data type)
	1989	5.5	National statistics (census)	1989	74.6	National statistics (census)
Albania....................	2011	7.9	DHS (survey)	2011	44.2	DHS (survey)
	1991	16.2	UNSD (census)	1991	35.9	UNSD (census)
Aruba	2010	14.1	National statistics (census)	2010	14.1	National statistics (census)
	1996	12.8	National statistics (census)	1996	37.7	National statistics (census)
Australia..................	2011	16.0	UNSD (census)	2011	28.9	UNSD (census)
	1995	7.6	FFS (survey)	1996	19.2	FFS (survey)
Austria	2010	21.1	OECD (registration)	2010	17.8	HFD (census and registration)
	1999	14.8	UNSD (census)	1999	57.0	UNSD (census)
Azerbaijan................	2009	12.3	UNSD (census)	2009	43.2	UNSD (census)
	1990	8.3	UNSD (census)	1990	63.8	UNSD (census)
Bahamas...................	2010	13.0	UNSD (census)	2010	40.7	UNSD (census)
	1989	6.6	UNSD (census)	1989	22.0	UNSD (census)
Belarus....................	2009	10.5	UNSD (census)	2009	10.5	UNSD (census)
	1990	12.8*	OECD (registration)			
Belgium	2000	15.2*	OECD (registration)			
	1991	10.2	UNSD (census)	1991	62.5	UNSD (census)
Brazil	2010	13.4	UNSD (census)	2010	36.8	UNSD (census)
	1998	8.2	FFS (Survey)	1998	10.2	FFS (Survey)
Bulgaria	2011	11.7	UNSD (census)	2011	8.4	UNSD (census)
	1991	15.9	UNSD (census)	1991	29.6	UNSD (census)
Canada	2007	18.9	HFD (census and registration)	2007	24.5	HFD (census and registration)
	1992	7.9	UNSD (census)			
Chile	2002	7.7	UNSD (census)			
	1991	9.4	UNSD (census)	1991	18.8	UNSD (census)
Croatia	2001	9.4	UNSD (census)	2001	21.5	UNSD (census)
	1991	5.5	UNSD (census)	1991	24.1	UNSD (census)
Czech Republic........	2011	7.1	UNSD (census)	2011	16.9	UNSD (census)
	1990	11.0§	OECD (registration)			
Denmark	2000	12.8§	OECD (registration)			
	1989	9.4	National Statistics (census)	1989	18.4	National Statistics (census)
Estonia....................	2011	10.2	UNSD (census)	2011	21.7	UNSD (census)
	1990	14.6	UNSD (census)	1990	24.1	UNSD (census)
Finland....................	2010	19.9	UNSD (census)	2010	28.0	UNSD (census)
	1990	8.1*	OECD (registration)			
France	2005	10.2*	OECD (registration)			
	1990	12.4*	OECD (registration)			
Greece.....................	2010	16.3*	OECD (registration)			
	1990	8.5	UNSD (census)	1990	19.0	UNSD (census)
Hungary	2011	12.0	UNSD (census)	2011	21.4	UNSD (census)
	1995	14.1§	OECD (registration)			
Ireland.....................	2011	19.0	UNSD (census)			
	1990	11.7*	OECD (registration)			
Italy........................	2009	20.1*	OECD (registration)			
	1992	9.2$^+$	National statistics	1992	27.5$^+$	National statistics (survey)
Japan	2010	19.2$^+$	National statistics	2010	22.9$^+$	National statistics (survey)

TABLE 3 CONT'D

	Childless			Three of More Children		
	Year	Percentage	Source (data type)	Year	Percentage	Source (data type)
	1995	12.2	FFS (Survey)	1995	16.3	FFS (Survey)
Lithuania..................	2011	8.4	UNSD (census)	2011	18.9	UNSD (census)
	1991	19.0	UNSD (census)	1991	20.4	UNSD (census)
Luxembourg.............	2001	15.4	UNSD (census)	2001	39.1	UNSD (census)
	1995	14.1	UNSD (census)	1995	33.8	UNSD (census)
Malta......................	2010	12.9	UNSD (census)	2010	25.6	UNSD (census)
	1990	3.7	UNSD (census)	1990	67.6	UNSD (census)
Mauritius.................	2011	4.5	UNSD (census)	2011	31.7	UNSD (census)
	1990	11.3*	OECD (registration)			
Netherlands.............	2010	18.3*	OECD (registration)			
	1990	9.7*	OECD (registration)			
Norway	2005	12.1*	OECD (registration)			
	1990	10.9*	OECD (registration)			
Poland	2010	15.5	OECD (registration)			
	1995	11.0*	OECD (registration)			
Portugal...................	2010	4.0	OECD (registration)			
	1990	3.6	UNSD (census)	1990	86.2	UNSD (census)
Republic of Korea....	2005	6.8	UNSD (census)	2005	13.6	UNSD (census)
Republic of	1989	9.2	UNSD (census)	1989	32.0	UNSD (census)
Moldova	2004	5.5	UNSD (census)	2004	30.3	UNSD (census)
	1992	9.7	UNSD (census)	1992	33.5	UNSD (census)
Romania...................	2002	10.5	UNSD (census)	2002	27.2	UNSD (census)
	1989	8.1	UNSD (census)	1989	16.7	UNSD (census)
Russian Federation...	2010	7.6	UNSD (census)	2010	12.0	UNSD (census)
	1991	10.7	UNSD (census)	1991	68.4	UNSD (census)
Saint Lucia..............	2001	9.8	UNSD (census)	2001	60.0	UNSD (census)
	1990	15.5	UNSD (census)	1990	40.4	UNSD (census)
Singapore................	2010	23.1	UNSD (census)	2010	22.8	UNSD (census)
	1990	9.9§	OECD(registration)			
Slovakia	2011	10.0	UNSD (census)			
	1991	9.4	UNSD (census)	1991	18.5	UNSD (census)
Slovenia	2002	7.0	UNSD (census)	2002	16.3	UNSD (census)
	1995	10.1§	OECD (registration)			
Spain	2011	21.6	UNSD (census)			
	1995	13.7§	OECD (registration)			
Sweden....................	2005	20.0§	OECD (registration)			
	1990	3.9	UNSD (census)	1990	61.1	UNSD (census)
Thailand..................	2005	11.4	UNSD (census)	2005	21.2	UNSD (census)
	1994	4.8	UNSD (census)	1994	29.8	UNSD (census)
TFYR Macedonia	2002	6.0	UNSD (census)	2002	28.8	UNSD (census)
	1989	7.2	UNSD (census)	1989	17.8	UNSD (census)
Ukraine	2007	5.4	DHS (survey)	2007	10.3	DHS (survey)
	1997	9.4	DHS (survey)	1997	72.0	DHS (survey)
Viet Nam.................	2002	8.4	DHS (survey)	2002	60.6	DHS (survey)

Note: DHS is Demographic and Health Surveys, FFS is Fertility and Family Surveys, HFD is the Human Fertility Database (a joint project of the Max Planck Institute for Demographic Research and the Vienna Institute of Demography), OCED is the Organisation for Economic Cooperation and Development, UNSD is the United Nations Statistics Division.
*Women aged 45 and over   §Women aged about 40   +Women aged 45-49.

	Around 1994			Latest available		
	Year	Percentage	Source	Year	Percentage	Source
Armenia	1995	15.2	UNSD	2009	35.3	UNSD
Australia.....................	1995	26.6	UNSD	2010	56.3	National statistics
Austria........................	1995	27.4	UNSD	2011	40.4	Eurostat
Azerbaijan..................	1996	4.0	UNSD	2012	15.5	Eurostat
Bahamas......................	1996	56.4	National Statistics	2009	61.5	UNSD
Belarus	1996	14.9	UNSD	2012	18.2	Eurostat
Belgium.......................	1992	13.6	UNSD	2011	50.0	Eurostat
Bosnia and Herzegovina	1991	7.9	UNSD	2010	10.8	UNSD
Bulgaria.......................	1995	25.7	UNSD	2012	57.4	Eurostat
Canada	1995	30.1	National statistics	2009	28.6	UNSD
Chile...........................	1995	40.5	UNSD	2009	67.4	UNSD
China, Hong Kong SAR	1995	4.7	UNSD	2009	8.3	UNSD
Costa Rica	1995	46.6	UNSD	2009	66.6	UNSD
Croatia........................	1995	7.5	UNSD	2012	15.4	Eurostat
Cyprus........................	1995	1.4	UNSD	2012	18.6	Eurostat
Czech Republic .... -	1995	15.6	UNSD	2012	43.3	Eurostat
Denmark......................	1995	46.1	UNSD	2012	50.6	Eurostat
Estonia	1995	44.1	UNSD	2012	58.4	Eurostat
Finland	1995	33.1	UNSD	2012	41.5	Eurostat
France.........................	1995	37.6	UNSD	2012	55.8	Eurostat
Georgia........................	1995	29.2	UNSD	2011	33.8	Eurostat
Germany......................	1995	16.1	UNSD	2012	34.5	Eurostat
Greece	1995	3.0	UNSD	2012	7.6	Eurostat
Hungary	1995	20.7	UNSD	2012	44.4	Eurostat
Ireland	1995	22.3	UNSD	2012	35.1	Eurostat
Italy	1995	8.1	UNSD	2011	24.5	Eurostat
Japan	1995	1.2	UNSD	2010	2.1	UNSD
Latvia	1995	29.9	UNSD	2012	45.0	Eurostat
Lithuania	1995	12.8	UNSD	2012	28.8	Eurostat
Luxembourg................	1995	13.1	UNSD	2012	37.1	Eurostat
Malta	1995	4.6	UNSD	2012	25.7	Eurostat
Mauritius.....................	1995	17.5	UNSD	2010	27.3	UNSD
Martinique...................	1992	66.0	UNSD	2007	73.0	UNSD
Netherlands	1995	15.5	UNSD	2011	46.6	Eurostat
Norway........................	1995	47.6	UNSD	2012	55.0	Eurostat
Poland	1995	9.5	UNSD	2012	22.3	Eurostat
Portugal.......................	1995	18.7	UNSD	2012	45.6	Eurostat
Puerto Rico..................	1994	41.9	UNSD	2008	61.2	UNSD
Republic of Moldova ..	1995	13.3	National Statistics	2012	22.4	Eurostat
Romania......................	1995	19.8	UNSD	2012	31.1	Eurostat
Russian Federation......	1995	21.1	UNSD	2011	24.8	Eurostat
Slovakia	1995	12.6	UNSD	2012	35.4	Eurostat
Slovenia	1995	29.8	UNSD	2012	27.6	Eurostat
Spain	1995	11.1	UNSD	2012	39.0	Eurostat
Sweden........................	1995	51.6	Eurostat	2012	54.5	Eurostat
Switzerland	1995	6.8	UNSD	2012	20.2	Eurostat
TFYR Macedonia........	1995	8.2	Eurostat	2011	11.6	Eurostat
Ukraine........................	1996	13.6	UNSD	2012	21.4	Eurostat
United Kingdom..........	1995	33.6	UNSD	2011	47.3	Eurostat

Region, country or area	Maximum fertility Year	TF	Onset of fertility transition Year	TF	Region, country or area	Maximum fertility Year	TF	Onset of fertility transition Year	TF
Eastern Africa									
Burundi	1988	7.6	2004	6.8	Rwanda	1979	8.4	1989	7.5
Comoros	1980	7.1	1986	6.4	Somalia	1997	7.7	2010	6.9
Djibouti	1972	6.8	1989	6.1	South Sudan	1975	6.9	1999	6.2
Eritrea	1955	7.0	1996	6.2	Uganda	1969	7.1	2008	6.3
Ethiopia	1984	7.4	1999	6.7	United Rep. of Tanzania	1961	6.8	1992	6.1
Kenya	1966	8.1	1982	7.3	Zambia	1973	7.4	1987	6.7
Madagascar	1971	7.3	1980	6.5	Zimbabwe	1972	7.4	1983	6.6
Malawi	1980	7.6	1991	6.9					
Mayotte	1975	8.0	1985	7.1					
Mozambique	1966	6.6	1996	5.9					
Western Africa									
Benin	1981	7.0	1996	6.3	Mali	1986	7.1		
Burkina Faso	1983	7.2	2003	6.4	Mauritania	1965	6.8	1987	6.1
Côte d'Ivoire	1973	7.9	1984	7.1	Niger	1985	7.8		
Gambia	1979	6.3			Nigeria	1980	6.8	2000	6.1
Ghana	1969	7.0	1984	6.2	Senegal	1976	7.5	1990	6.6
Guinea	1986	6.6	2000	5.9	Sierra Leone	1980	7.1	1993	6.3
Guinea-Bissau	1950	8.5	1952	7.6	Togo	1976	7.3	1989	6.5
Liberia	1981	7.0	1994	6.2					
Middle Africa									
Angola	1965	7.4	2005	6.7	Dem. Rep. of the Congo	1995	7.3	2008	6.5
Cameroon	1984	6.7	1995	6.0	Equatorial Guinea	1993	5.9	2008	5.3
Central African Rep	1982	6.0	2002	5.3	Gabon	1983	5.7	1994	5.1
Chad	1996	7.4	2010	6.6	Sao Tome and Principe	1975	6.5	1986	5.9
Congo	1975	6.3	1986	5.7					
Northern and Southern Africa									
Lesotho	1956	5.9	1986	5.2	Sudan	1975	6.9	1989	6.2
Namibia	1975	6.7	1985	5.9	Swaziland	1971	6.9	1987	6.2
Asia									
Afghanistan	1997	7.9	2005	6.9	Philippines	1950	7.4	1966	6.7
Iraq	1950	8.1	1972	7.2	State of Palestine	1965	8.1	1981	7.2
Jordan	1965	8.1	1980	7.3	Tajikistan	1970	6.9	1977	6.0
Lao People's Dem. Rep.	1984	6.4	1994	5.6	Timor-Leste	2000	7.1	2009	6.4
Pakistan	1975	6.6	1991	5.9	Yemen	1984	9.2	1993	8.1
Latin America and the Caribbean									
Bolivia	1955	6.8	1976	6.0	Haiti	1960	6.3	1988	5.7
French Guiana	1965	5.1	1971	4.5	Honduras	1955	7.5	1976	6.8
Guatemala	1950	7.2	1961	6.5					
Oceania									
Micronesia, Fed. States	1950	7.3	1977	6.5	Solomon Islands	1974	7.3	1983	6.4
Papua New Guinea	1962	6.3	1981	5.6	Tonga	1960	7.4	1967	6.6
Samoa	1960	7.7	1974	6.9	Vanuatu	1950	7.7	1964	6.8

Source: United Nations (2013a).
NOTE: TF is Total fertility.

Percentage decline in total fertility between 1994 and 2010

Eastern Africa	Percentage	Middle Africa	Percentage	Western Africa	Percentage
Burundi	14.4	Angola	11.9	Benin	21.0
Comoros	6.4	Cameroon	17.5	Burkina Faso	14.7
Djibouti	35.0	Central African Rep.	17.7	Côte d'Ivoire	16.8
Eritrea	21.8	Chad	11.1	Gambia	4.3
Ethiopia	30.4	Congo	1.9	Ghana	21.5
Kenya	14.0	Dem. Rep. of the Congo	14.0	Guinea	18.8
Madagascar	23.3	Equatorial Guinea	12.9	Guinea-Bissau	20.1
Malawi	13.8	Gabon	17.0	Liberia	19.1
Mayotte	17.2	Sao Tome and Principe	14.8	Mali	1.9
Mozambique	10.3			Mauritania	16.0
Rwanda	24.5	*Northern Africa*	*Percentage*	Niger	2.4
Somalia	9.8	Sudan	21.3	Nigeria	4.5
South Sudan	20.9			Senegal	18.1
Tanzania	8.7	*Southern Africa*	*Percentage*	Sierra Leone	21.0
Uganda	12.6	Lesotho	30.5	Togo	17.9
Zambia	6.9	Namibia	31.5		
Zimbabwe	18.3	Swaziland	29.3		

Asia	Percentage	Latin America and the Caribbean	Percentage	Oceania	Percentage
Afghanistan	27.4	Bolivia	28.0	Micronesia	26.6
Iraq	23.6	French Guiana	21.9	Papua New Guinea	15.6
Jordan	28.4	Guatemala	25.3	Samoa	9.9
Lao People's Dem. Rep.	41.3	Haiti	33.0	Solomon Islands	20.5
Pakistan	37.6	Honduras	33.4	Tonga	13.0
Philippines	22.3			Vanuatu	26.7
State of Palestine	34.2				
Tajikistan	19.7				
Timor-Leste	-1.8				
Yemen	42.6				

Source: United Nations (2013a).

	Mean age at first marriage		Mean age at first birth		Source
	Year	Age	Year	Age	
Benin................................	1996	18.7	1996	19.8	DHS 1996
	2011-12	19.3	2011-12	20.3	DHS 2011-12
Bolivia................................	1994	20.6	1994	21.1	DHS 1994
	2008	21.1	2008	21.2	DHS 2008
Burkina Faso........................	1993	17.5	1993	19.0	DHS 1993
	2010	17.9	2010	19.4	DHS 2010
Cameroon............................. .	1998	18.0	1998	19.0	DHS 1998
	2011	19.0	2011	19.7	DHS 2011
Chad..................................	1996-97	15.9	1996-97	18.2	DHS 1996-97
	2004	16.0	2004	18.2	DHS 2004
Cote d'Ivoire........................	1998-99	19.7	1998-99	19.2	DHS 1998-99
	2011-12	20.5	2011-12	19.8	DHS 2011-12
Eritrea	1995	17.4	1995	20.9	DHS 1995
	2002	18.4	2002	20.6	DHS 2002
Gabon................................	2000	20.4	2000	18.7	DHS 2000
	2012	22.1	2012	20.3	DHS 2012
Ghana................................	1998	19.6	1993	20.3	DHS 1998
	2008	21.0	2008	21.8	DHS 2008
Guatemala............................	1995	19.1	1995	20.2	DHS 1995
	2008-09	19.4	2008-09	20.5	RHS 2008-09
Guinea................................	1999	16.5	1999	18.6	DHS 1999
	2012	17.4	2012	18.9	DHS 2012
Haiti	1994-95	20.5	1995	21.9	DHS 1994-95
	2012	22.1	2012	22.7	DHS-MICS 2012
Jordan................................	1990	21.2	1990	23.0	DHS 1990
	2012	23.0	2012	24.7	DHS 2012
Kenya................................	1998	20.2	1998	19.6	DHS 1998
	2008-09	20.2	2008-09	19.8	DHS 2008-9
Madagascar..........................	1997	18.9	1997	19.8	DHS 1997
	2008-09	18.4	2008-09	19.5	DHS 2008-09
Malawi................................	1992	17.7	1992	18.7	DHS 1992
	2010	17.9	2010	18.9	DHS 2010
Mali..................................	1995-96	16.8	1995-96	18.6	DHS 1995-96
	2012-13	17.4	2012-13	18.8	DHS 2012-13
Mozambique	1997	17.3	1997	18.7	DHS 1997
	2011	18.3	2011	18.9	DHS 2011
Namibia.............................			1992	21.2	DHS 1992
			2006-07	21.4	DHS 2006-07
Niger	1992	14.9	1992	17.8	DHS 1992
	2012	15.9	2012	18.1	DHS 2012

TABLE 7 CONT'D

	Mean age at first marriage		Mean age at first birth		Source
	Year	Age	Year	Age	
Nigeria................................	1990	17.2	1990	19.6	DHS 1990
	2013	18.6	2013	20.3	DHS 2013
Pakistan...............................	1990-91	18.9	1990-91	22.0	DHS 1990-91
	2012-13	20.9	2012-13	23.4	DHS 2012-13
Philippines.	1993	22.0	1993	23.1	DHS 1993
	2013	22.1	2013	23.0	DHS 2013
Rwanda	1992	20.9	1992	22.0	DHS 1992
	2010	22.3	2010	22.9	DHS 2010
Senegal................................	1992-93	16.8	1992-93	19.3	DHS 1992-93
	2010-11	19.9	2010-11	21.4	DHS 2010-11
Tajikistan	1995	21.1	1995	21.8	UNECE (registration)
	2010	22.5	2009	23.6	UNECE (registration)
Tanzania..............................	1996	18.7	1996	19.4	DHS 1996
	2010	18.9	2010	19.6	DHS 2010
Uganda................................	1995	17.8	1995	18.9	DHS 1995
	2011	18.2	2011	18.9	DHS 2011
Zambia................................	1996	18.4	1996	19.0	DHS 1996
	2007	18.7	2007	19.2	DHS 2007
Zimbabwe	1994	19.3	1994	19.7	DHS 1994
	2010-11	19.9	2010-11	20.5	DHS 2010-11

NOTE: DHS is Demographic and Health Surveys, MICS is Multiple Indicator Cluster Survey, RHS is Reproductive Health Survey, UNECE is United Nations Economic Commission for Europe.